PENGUIN B

# natural children's health

PENELOPE SACH is Australia's leading practitioner of naturopathic, homeopathic and herbal medicine. She runs a highly successful clinic in Sydney and produces her own range of organically grown herbal teas. Her most recent books include *Natural Woman*, *Natural Men's Health* and *Detox*.

For more about Penelope Sach,
visit www.penelopesach.com.au

Other titles by Penelope Sach

*The Little Book of Wellbeing*
*Take Care of Yourself*
*Healing and Cleansing with Herbal Tea*
*Detox*
*Natural Woman*
*Natural Men's Health*

# natural children's health

**PENELOPE SACH**

PENGUIN BOOKS

*This book is not intended to replace or supersede professional medical advice. Neither the author nor the publisher may be held responsible for claims resulting from information contained in this book.*

PENGUIN BOOKS

Published by the Penguin Group
Penguin Group (Australia)
250 Camberwell Road, Camberwell, Victoria 3124, Australia
(a division of Pearson Australia Group Pty Ltd)
Penguin Group (USA) Inc.
375 Hudson Street, New York, New York 10014, USA
Penguin Group (Canada)
10 Alcorn Avenue, Toronto, Ontario, Canada M4V 3B2
(a division of Pearson Penguin Canada Inc.)
Penguin Books Ltd
80 Strand, London WC2R 0RL, England
Penguin Ireland
25 St Stephen's Green, Dublin 2, Ireland
(a division of Penguin Books Ltd)
Penguin Books India Pvt Ltd
11 Community Centre, Panchsheel Park, New Delhi – 110 017, India
Penguin Group (NZ)
Cnr Airborne and Rosedale Roads, Albany, Auckland, New Zealand
(a division of Pearson New Zealand Ltd)
Penguin Books (South Africa) (Pty) Ltd
24 Sturdee Avenue, Rosebank, Johannesburg 2196, South Africa

Penguin Books Ltd, Registered Offices: 80 Strand, London, WC2R 0RL, England

First published by Penguin Group (Australia), a division of Pearson Australia Group Pty Ltd, 2005

1 3 5 7 9 10 8 6 4 2

Copyright © Penelope Sach 2005

The moral right of the author has been asserted

All rights reserved. Without limiting the rights under copyright reserved above, no part of this publication may be reproduced, stored in or introduced into a retrieval system, or transmitted, in any form or by any means (electronic, mechanical, photocopying, recording or otherwise), without the prior written permission of both the copyright owner and the above publisher of this book.

Design by David Altheim © Penguin Group (Australia)
Cover photograph © Julie Anne Renouf
Author photograph © Louise Lister
Typeset in ITC Legacy Serif by Post Pre-press Group, Brisbane, Queensland
Printed and bound in Australia by McPherson's Printing Group, Maryborough, Victoria

National Library of Australia
Cataloguing-in-Publication data:

Sach, Penelope.
Natural children's health.

Includes index.
ISBN 0 14 300265 1.

1. Children – Health and hygiene – Australia – Handbooks, manuals, etc. 2. Naturopathy – Australia. I. Title.

613.0432

www.penguin.com.au

# Contents

|    | *Introduction*            | 1   |
|----|---------------------------|-----|
| 1  | The immune system         | 9   |
| 2  | Asthma                    | 24  |
| 3  | Earaches and tonsillitis  | 36  |
| 4  | The brain                 | 48  |
| 5  | The anxious child         | 68  |
| 6  | Skin conditions           | 86  |
| 7  | The digestive system      | 95  |
| 8  | The four seasons          | 108 |
| 9  | Nutrition and weight control | 117 |
| 10 | A child's healthy diet    | 131 |
| 11 | Common childhood issues   | 146 |
|    | *How to buy supplements*  | 153 |
|    | *Conclusion*              | 157 |
|    | *Index*                   | 160 |

I would like to dedicate *Natural Children's Health* to the many beautiful children I have treated over the years, who have profoundly touched me with their inner wisdom and insight into the spiritual understandings beyond ourselves.

# Introduction

*Natural Children's Health* has come about from the countless requests I have received over the years from frustrated parents whose children I have had the pleasure of helping regain health and vitality. Through simple changes to diet, lifestyle or added nutritional supplements, these parents have seen their children freed from the cycles of winter flus, skin ailments, poor concentration and mood swings. The parents have in return gained stronger and healthier children, with the freedom of not having to use pharmaceutical medication unnecessarily.

When I began practice as a naturopath in 1988 my main clientele were mothers who were stressed and frustrated with not only their own health but the general health ailments of their children. At that time I wanted to specialise in children's health, because there was very little on offer for parents seeking the guidance of natural health principles when treating their children's needs and illnesses. There were also very few health food stores that catered to these families.

I had been very fortunate to study at the Southern Cross Herbal Medicine School in Sydney, run by Denis Stewart, who was widely regarded as the master of herbal medicine in Australia. During my time studying with Denis, I gained immeasurable academic knowledge and hands-on experience through observing plants in the wild and making plant medicine from herbs such as nettle and mullein.

I continued to study everything I could find that would give me a deeper understanding of children's health. I learned about the use of herbal medicine in relation to birthing and rearing children. This knowledge, which women have passed down through the ages, is incredibly rich, even when compared to the knowledge and advances we have achieved through science and Western medical practices.

In 1989 I had the pleasure of travelling to Bali and Jakarta, where I saw and compared the foods of this region to those of Australia and was able to work with some herbalists in Jakarta who were specialising in pregnancy, childbirth and children's health. I observed the basic diets of the children and the ways in which the children's behavioural patterns were affected by the local foods and herbs they ate, and I studied the changes in children's behaviour and the developing health problems that occurred when these children were introduced to a Western diet.

During this time I continued to research the art of blending plants, by which I mean blending the empirical knowledge of plant 'synergy' with the scientific knowledge of plant healing. Put simply, some herbs work much better when they are blended with other plants. I learned the methods of philosophy and blending herbs through the European–Western–American art of healing where diet, lifestyle and plants are all an aid to trigger the natural forces of healing. The Chinese and Ayurvedic methods of philosophy and plant healing also have their important place, and now all these systems use plants grown all over the world; these plants can be blended according to the patient's symptoms, ailments, personality and lifestyle.

The marriage of ancient uses of plants with scientific pharmacology has been a truly remarkable breakthrough of the twenty-first century. Science is now showing us that practices from centuries ago – such as the ancient Romans' practice of reaping the benefits of goat's milk, myrrh and honey; the use of medieval 'herbal concoctions' made from nettle (blood cleanser), red clover (anti-cancer herb), lemon balm (nervine herb) and thyme (natural antiseptic); the eighteenth century use of Hawthorn Berry (heart herb), chamomile, sage and marjoram in the United Kingdom and United States; and practices of the monks in China who have for centuries used ginkgo biloba (memory herb) and ginsengs (for physical and mental stamina) – can be adapted and continued as we move forward. Now more than ever we are recognising the vital role plants play in natural medicine.

In both Western society and the discipline of natural medicine studies, there is a tendency to give a disease a long and fancy name. But through experience I have discovered that however complicated the name is, accurate diagnosis is all about observation and information. The observation of the whole patient needs to be considered. This is where I believe that natural medicine has a great strength: when considering a child's illness, the whole child is taken into account, including socio-economic background, daily food intake, school background and performance, colour and quality of the skin, allergies and mood swings.

For me, the key word in treating children and their ailments is 'building'. Build their resistance to disease through the right foods. Build their mind through feeding their body complete foods that contain the vitamins and minerals so essential to the growing child. Build their confidence through routine and positive thoughts and actions. Build their love of the planet through respect and admiration for all living things. Build their love of humankind through kind words and deeds.

We are only at the beginning of our scientific knowledge about how our children's brains work and develop. But we do know if we feed our children healthy, complete foods (whole foods that have not been stripped of the outer shell where the nutrients lie, and have no added colouring or preservatives), avoid drugs where possible and give children plenty of exercise and sunlight with love wrapped in between, then we will be breeding the world's – and our future's – strength.

Enjoy this book and use it to gain knowledge and familiarity with children's health issues. Try to persist with the foods and supplements recommended (and make sure you administer the supplements after your child has eaten). Nothing happens overnight with natural healing, but over a surprisingly short time the results can be quite spectacular. Remember that when you take the time to be patient and consistent with your child, you are 'building' their living cells.

In this book I do not deal with infants; my advice is aimed at children between the ages of five and twelve. I have tried to cover the most important childhood illnesses that can be successfully treated at an early stage with preventative natural medicine. Naturopathic treatment in children is especially useful when dealing with allergies, hyperactivity, growth problems, learning, stomach upsets, common colds, coughs and flus.

When dealing with symptoms, I have purposely avoided using complex medical names; I have opted instead for descriptive names for certain early symptoms. All too often I see parents and doctors trying to fit a child's symptoms into a 'disease disorder', when the problem may simply be a passing disturbance of the natural equilibrium of their health and development. As a naturopath and herbalist, I follow the principle of using the body's own natural forces to heal, repair and make well. Therefore, foods, herbs and vitamins are always the frontrunner to any healing regime. This is especially important with children, whose developing systems are much more delicate than those of adults. I advise you to use the information in this book about how to naturally deal with your child's problems *before* taking your child to the doctor's surgery.

The same approach applies to each chapter of this book. You will see that the symptoms of some minor problems must be addressed by changing diet and administering herbs. Herbs (plants) are very effective for nutrition and healing. Herbs as commonplace as parsley, ginger, chamomile, thyme and peppermint stimulate the body to naturally heal, and they can also stimulate cell tissue, which aids healing when dealing with deeper problems such as a lowered immune system and a frayed nervous system. Herbs also have a natural affinity to assist in destroying chemical pollutants in the blood, which we and our children are exposed to on a daily basis.

A doctor should always be consulted if your child shows no improvement after a short time (this will be more specifically discussed in each chapter). It is perfectly acceptable for a doctor and a naturopath to work side by side for the benefit of your child's health. Through my studies and practice I have come to realise how profound our wisdom can be if we acknowledge both strands of medicine: the use of traditional healing plants as preventive medicine as well as for healing certain illnesses; and the use of Western medicine, when needed, for major illness and diseases.

Pharmaceutical medicine can successfully run alongside appropriate herbal medicine or supplements. This book will give you basic guidelines for dosages of appropriate and safe herbs. It is always advisable to consult with a naturopath for any unusual cases or where different dosages might be indicated for your child. (That is, if you are not happy with your child's progress, a higher dose may be appropriate for a short time, and here it would be advisable to consult with a naturopath.)

To all those parents who have so patiently waited for this book and for those parents who are in need of basic guidelines for their children's health without frills and complicated explanations, may *Natural Children's Health* be a blessing for you. My final words to you are: never give up, persevere with nutritional values of fresh foods, and try the suggestions in this book – they have worked for thousands of children. The rewards you reap will be your proud satisfaction in a happy and healthy child.

# 1
# The immune system

The immune system is a very intricate and complex system. Put simply, it is responsible for making the white blood cells in the body (in areas called the 'lymph glands', found in the neck area, under the arms and the groin area). White blood cells are our natural 'fighter army cells' that attack the foreign bodies such as bacteria and viruses that we pick up in our journey through life. This system needs to be kept in tune; otherwise it becomes run down, clogged or fatigued. For example, if your child has caught numerous colds, their white cell count works very hard to combat the bacteria or virus. If the immune system is continually bombarded with viruses, it never has time to make fresh white blood cells, and hence the endless cycle of colds and flus can continue. Rest, fresh air, fresh food and natural healing plants are prescribed in these cases to assist the body to repair vitality and make new cells. We often know when the first signs of a lowered immune system kick in by seeing our child's swollen tonsils or neck glands, or in a virus situation a red raw throat with swollen glands under the ear area.

So boosting the immune system is the first step to recovery and prevention in children's health. Try the following program to help your child gain strength and vitality.

## ✱ Boosting the immune system

The following immunity-boosting program focuses on your child's diet, and is especially effective if started before the difficult seasons begin – if your child is prone to coughs, colds and flus, start well before winter; if they are prone to allergies, start well before spring; if food allergies are the issue, then right now is the right time! If your child suffers from a severe cough, cold, flu or other illness, they may need an antibiotic, so speak to your doctor. If antibiotics are prescribed, it is even more essential for your child to follow this program to boost their immune system during and after the illness.

- Protein is an essential component in repairing damaged cell tissue and building new cells for the immune system. Feed your child different forms of protein twice daily: fish, lean red meats, eggs, nuts and legumes are all complete proteins and can be varied (see the child's healthy diet in chapter 10). Cheese and milk (soy or rice milk if your child is allergic to dairy) are also forms of protein.

- Fish contains vitamin A and fatty acids essential for a strong immune system. Deep-sea fish such as salmon, mackerel, sardines and tuna are especially good because they contain omega 3 for building the lining of the mucous membrane that runs through the sinus passages and lungs. (Ensure any fish you serve your child is thoroughly deboned.) If your child resists, try coating the fillet in rice crumbs and frying it lightly in olive oil and butter.

- Omega 6 oils are also essential. Omega 6 comes from vegetable oil, particularly flaxseed. You can buy a combination liquid (omega 3 and 6 oils) – try 1 teaspoon twice a day, especially throughout winter.

- Fruits are high in vitamin C and bioflavonoids, which build the white cell count (critical for good immunity) and strengthen the body against viruses. Orange fruits are rich in antioxidants, which strengthen immunity; try oranges, mangoes, peaches and apricots. Watermelon, pineapple, grapes and berries are also high in vitamin C and antioxidants. For younger children, it may help to cut fruit into small portions or animal figures, making the fruit more interesting and easy to chew.

- Avoid fruit juices containing additives and preservatives, which can be too acidic for children with tender digestive systems. Stick to freshly squeezed juice diluted with water, or replace juices with stewed fruits.

- Eliminate refined sugars, white flours, cordials, fizzy drinks, preservatives and additives from your child's diet. These substances overload the liver (the organ that filters the blood) and can affect the balance of chemicals in the brain, skin irritations and asthma.

- Make sure your child has plenty of vegetables each day. Orange vegetables are rich in antioxidants; try sweet potato, pumpkin and carrots. Green vegetables are essential for iron and other nutrients. Your child may be resistant to spinach, broccoli, zucchini or lettuce, but try a little each day or hide it by mashing it into potato or mixing it through vegetable soups. Try sweetening vegetable soups with pumpkin.

- Zinc is essential for strong immunity. Pumpkin seeds are high in zinc, but children often don't like these seeds unless you can incorporate them in a fine powder and sprinkle over cereal. Otherwise, ask your herbalist or naturopath for a multivitamin that contains zinc.

# Supplements

I recommend the following supplements in the winter months.

- Half a teaspoon of echinacea glycetract (a non-alcohol-based herbal supplement you can obtain from a herbalist) dissolved in milk, juice or water once a day if your child is well; if your child is ill, give two to three times a day.

- Give 1 teaspoon a day of a liquid iron tonic based on fruits high in vitamin C. You can find this at your health food store.

- If symptoms persist, a tonic can be given made from herbs: Cat's claw, echinacea and andrographis (see the following section on coughs, colds and flus).

> ### Glycetracts
> Glycetracts or glycerites are liquid preparations made using glycerol and water instead of ethanol and water. They are useful where the active components of a herb are water soluble. Not all herbs are ideal for this. Generally they taste better and are sweeter than alcohol-based medicine.

# ✳ Coughs, colds and flus

Most parents are well aware of the onset of a cough, cold or flu in their child. The illness generally begins with a sniffle, which can develop into a blocked or runny nose. If your child has a runny nose discharging white phlegm and the discharge turns green or yellow, this often indicates an infection in the nose or sinus passages, and it must not be left untreated. Take your child to your doctor, who can examine your child and advise accordingly. (If your child suffers from a year-round blocked or runny nose and seems to have a slight wheeze or bronchial problem, refer to chapter 2 on asthma.)

The phlegm (or mucous drip) in a runny nose can aggravate the child's upper respiratory system and cause a nasty sore or bacterial throat. If left unchecked this can often turn into a bacterial infection and drip into the chest, causing bronchitis or aggravating asthma. In adults we often refer to this as sinusitis, but with children up to the age of twelve, the symptoms are generally treated as an upper respiratory infection or a bronchial infection, particularly if the bacteria or virus gets into the lungs.

# Preventative program

- Avoid heavy, starchy foods, such as breads, pastries and cakes, for the duration of a blocked or runny nose, and cut back on dairy products and sweets. These foods can slow the body down, and in some children can aggravate the production of mucous. It is always better to stay with lighter foods, such as cooked and raw vegetables, fruits and proteins. Give your child vegetable soups and fresh fruits, and follow the child's healthy diet set out in chapter 10.

- Echinacea is a wonderful herb for avoiding and combating a blocked or runny nose. For children aged five to twelve, give 1 teaspoon of echinacea glycetract twice a day for three to four weeks before winter. (Children often prefer the 'sweeter' taste of non-alcohol-based medicine and it never upsets the stomach.)

- Organic loose-leaf peppermint herbal tea with honey is very good in the weeks leading up to winter. The menthol oil in the leaf assists the clearance of phlegm, and the hot steam from the tea stimulates the clearance of a stuffy nose.

# Treatment

If your child does not show signs of recovery in the early stages of sinusitis, they may need a change of medicine from your naturopath. If the infection still does not improve after four to seven days, your child should see a doctor in case an antibiotic needs to be given alongside the natural medicine.

- Rest and long sleeps are essential, so keep your child home from school when they are suffering from a cold or the flu.

- Keep your child's fluid intake high to avoid dehydration, especially when they have a minor temperature and are sweating. Soups are ideal. Watermelon eaten whole or juiced helps prevent dehydration, and most children love the taste. Freshly squeezed lemon juice (a quarter to a half a lemon) with warm water, 1 teaspoon of dark natural honey and a sprinkle of cinnamon is wonderful.

- To reduce a temperature, soothe the throat and respiratory tract and stop dehydration during respiratory problems in children over the age of six, try a herbal tea made from equal parts of loose-leaf organic peppermint and elderflower, a pinch of cinnamon and a tiny sprinkle of ginger powder. Make up enough to last for a few days. Add 1 teaspoon of the dried mixture to 2 cups of boiling water, then add 1 teaspoon of honey and serve the tea hot to your child every two to three hours.

- You can use an echinacea spray two to three times a day to soothe the back of the throat.

- A eucalyptus–peppermint (menthol) inhalant, or a pH-balanced salt water spray – both obtainable from a pharmacy – are wonderful in helping to clear a blocked nose. Your child can carry one in their pocket or schoolbag.

> ### Echinacea
>
> There are three species of echinacea (commonly known as purple cone) that are used medicinally. *Echinacea purpurea* is the most cultivated and widely used. Various parts of the plant – root, leaf,

> flower and seed – can be used. Information about the use of echinacea first came from native American tribes. Echinacea is classed as an immunostimulant and is beneficial for the prophylaxis (prevention) of infections in general. Echinacea enhances resistance to infections, particularly in the upper respiratory system. There is no evidence to suggest that long-term use of echinacea will have an adverse effect on immune function.

# Supplements

- Three weeks before cold winter weather sets in, give your child a daily supplement of 100–200 mg of vitamin C with bioflavonoids. You can buy this in a powder for children – which is usually far superior and a higher dose than chewable tablets – and mix the powder into juice or a milkshake. If diarrhoea occurs, lower the dose. Don't worry – you cannot overdose or hurt your child with vitamin C.

- Omega 3 and omega 6 oils are essential. Try 1 teaspoon twice a day (especially throughout winter) of an oil from your health food store.

- If your child is prone to upper respiratory flus and colds (which are bacterial in origin; coloured phlegm is usually present in these cases), use an echinacea herb extract made from a glycetract base. (If you are unsure whether your child is suffering from a bacterial infection, check with your doctor.) If your child is prone to viral infections (symptoms include ear infections, raspy coughs and general debility; and there will usually not be a discharge or phlegm), incorporate echinacea (*Echinacea purpurea*) with anti-viral herbs such as Cats claw (*Uncaria tomentose*) and immunity-enhancing herbs such as *Andrographis paniculate*; this latter (traditional Ayurvedic) herb increases antibodies in non-specific immune deficiency illnesses such as the common cold. Both herbs can be bought in tonics from your health food store, or ask your naturopath. For children aged five to eight, give 2 ml once or twice a day; for older children, give 4 ml twice a day.

▦ A natural iron supplement before winter is important for children because iron is essential for building immunity, and many of our children are anaemic (they have low iron levels) due to poor nutrition and eating habits and our decreasing consumption of red meat. Natural, pleasant-tasting iron tonics made from fruits and berries are widely available. Half to 1 teaspoon once a day throughout winter can help prevent children from developing chronic respiratory problems. Ask your health food store for a high-quality liquid iron tonic suitable for your child's age.

---

### An old and useful remedy for a barking cough

Preheat your oven to moderate. Cut a white onion into quarters and place on a baking tray. Drizzle 2 tablespoons of honey over the onion and then bake for 20 minutes. Siphon off the syrup and give it to your child every 10 minutes. This syrup is soothing and helps calm severe coughs. The onion has wonderful antibiotic and antibacterial attributes that are short-lasting but will assist even if your child is on antibiotics.

### Vaccination

Throughout my years in private practice I have advised parents on the subject of vaccination as I would on the subject of contraception: I point out all the pros and cons and let them decide.

I am a great advocate of raising a child's immune system. If a child is to have a vaccination, the immune system should be strong; but if a child is not to be vaccinated, then the immune system absolutely must be strong. Either way, the following herbs are vital for boosting a child's white cell count and strengthening the immune system against bacterial and viral infection.

If you choose to vaccinate your child, I recommend that you make the time of vaccination for when the child is well – if possible, wait for the summer months, when flus and colds are less prevalent. I set a child on the following program for two to four weeks before vaccinations.

- One multivitamin tablet each day.
- An equal mix of herbs *Andrographis paniculate* and Cats claw (*Uncaria tomentose*): for children

over the age of five, give 20 drops twice a day.
- Cod liver oil with natural vitamin A protects against immunisation reactions such as fever and nausea: for children over the age of five, give half a teaspoon twice a day; for children aged over six, give 1 teaspoon once a day.
- To relieve side effects and possible fevers caused by vaccinations, give your child the homoeopathic Thuja in 30 potency (your naturopath can explain the various levels of dilution for you): 2 drops into the mouth twice on the day before the vaccination, and again a few hours before going to the doctor.

# 2
# Asthma

Asthma occurs for many reasons, and in my experience natural medical treatments can be very supportive in preventing attacks in children. The most common triggers of asthma attacks in both children and adults are common colds and allergies. It is therefore very important to keep your child's immune system strong (see chapter 1) and to obtain a thorough knowledge of your child's particular allergies to airborne irritants and food. I always encourage parents to consult their doctor to properly diagnose asthma in their child, because doctors have the medical equipment for testing lung capacity and can carry out simple tests for food allergies.

The most common allergies to aggravate asthma in children are dust mites. These little critters are microscopic in size and live in the dust of carpets, curtains, bedding or wherever there is warm and cosy place for them to be. I always advise my clients who suffer from asthma to keep dust at bay as much as possible. If practicable, have floorboards (not carpet) in your home, and regularly air out pillows and bedding. Your local asthma society can often give excellent support and tips on keeping dust mites to a minimum.

Food allergies can be checked by a test called a Rast test, performed by a doctor, which is a simple scratch test on the child's arm.

In my consulting experience I have found that asthma can be treated very effectively by eliminating certain high-response allergy foods. An allergy food can be one item or a group of foods that the body does not correctly break down or that causes a histamine reaction such as hives and rashes; in some extreme cases, this reaction can cause hyperventilation and, in very rare cases, death. A child may not be allergic to a food all their life. As they grow they can simply become food sensitive and show mild symptoms. You can often identify an allergy food by removing it from your child's diet for six weeks, then returning the food to the diet every three to four days and observing your child's symptoms. The foods most likely to trigger asthma attacks are wheat, whole dairy, preservatives and additives, because these foods and chemicals can lower the immune response in susceptible children. In controlling the symptoms of asthma, concerted effort needs to be made to eliminate each of these until you are sure which your child is allergic to.

After your child has avoided the problem foods for three to six months, you can test your child very gently and carefully, one food at a time, to gauge reaction. If the asthma flares up again, remove all trace of the problem food. It can be gradually reintroduced later when the immune system has recovered.

Another factor to consider if your child suffers from asthma is their emotional state. Asthma attacks can be brought on if your child is suffering from emotional problems caused by incidents at school or in the home. If this appears to be the case, talk to your child about these issues, or find a suitable counsellor to help your child through any difficulties.

Other elements that can cause asthma flare-ups in children include animal hair, particularly cat and horse hair; flowering trees and shrubs in your garden – check the trees in your garden for aggravating pollens, especially those that occur at the change of season, and check with an expert at your local asthma society to identify plants that have high levels of pollens; household sprays and cleaning agents, which can contain harmful ingredients; and air conditioning or extreme changes in temperature, particularly hot to cold, because the body loses vital heat, which can bring on asthma and bronchial problems.

Parents of asthmatic children need to be especially vigilant during spring and autumn, when airborne aggravators abound. At this time, an inflammation of the respiratory tract can occur very quickly, leading to asthma attacks. Pay special attention to diet and supplements during these times of the year.

## Treatment

From my observation, the longer a child has been following the correct diet and supplements, the fewer asthma attacks they have. They become stronger and happier in themselves. Sometimes children need some asthma medication from their doctor, and natural treatment can run alongside this medication.

- Follow the preventative program outlined for coughs, colds and flus (see page 16), but take particular care to start your child on this program at least a month before the change of seasons. Continue these supplements through winter, and give your child a break during summer.

- Take particular care with your child's diet. Regular meals and snacks for children are important to maintain energy – remember that children have smaller stomachs than adults and need to eat every three to four hours.

- Remove wheat, whole milk and all food additives and preservatives from your child's diet. This means no tinned foods or fizzy drinks. Use only rye or rice breads and cut out wheat pasta; use rice pasta instead. If you are avoiding dairy, try the alternatives of soy milk (preferably with added calcium), rice milk or goat's milk. As you remove these items from your child's diet, incorporate a whey protein powder concentrate – available from a health food store – to maintain the nutrients your child needs. You can add 1 tablespoon to a milkshake or sprinkle 2 teaspoons over cereal – children love it.

- Avoid pre-processed or sugary snacks – go for healthy snacks such as sandwiches filled with chicken, egg, ham or beef. Vary breads (not wheat breads) with dry biscuits such as Ryvita biscuits. Take care not to overload your child with sweets or chocolate, because they are very high in concentrated sugars and can often trigger an asthma attack. There are now sweets and jubes widely available that do not have colourings or additives, so try these for special occasions.

- Remove peanuts from your child's diet, because many children with asthma are allergic to them. Peanuts are a legume and contain a substance called vicilin, a protein that can often aggravate asthma-sensitive children. Observe your child after they have eaten nuts, and if you suspect that your child is allergic, eliminate nuts from their diet for six weeks.

- Organic dried fruits, such as apricots, pears and prunes, are a good snack. (If your child finds them unpalatable, soak them overnight to improve the softness and flavour.) Buy only organic dried fruit, because many dried fruits are sprayed with sulphur, which can cause an allergic reaction.

- Serve only fresh fruits and vegetables with proteins such as hormone- and chemical-free fish, chicken and red meat. If your child is vegetarian, include plenty of legumes, such as lima beans, adzuki beans and split peas. Regardless of whether your child is vegetarian, introduce them to these complete proteins in the forms of vegetable soups or in stews served with brown rice.

- Include soy yoghurt, rice milk and goat's milk in your child's diet. Goat's yoghurt is high in calcium, so find a good-quality yoghurt with added acidophilus (good bacteria that helps with children's digestion).

- Freshly squeezed orange and pineapple juices, and watermelon are very high in vitamin C. You may need to dilute these with water for younger children. Fresh berries and all orange fruits are high in antioxidants.

- Peppermint and lemongrass tea with honey is a great alternative to fizzy drinks. Iceblocks made from peppermint tea with honey are a great treat for children.

- Chicken broth and vegetable soups are an excellent way to maintain your child's nutritional and fluid intake. Often when children are unwell, they do not want to eat, so soup is a great way to encourage food and healing into their bodies.

## Supplements

- Omega 3 and 6 oils are essential for an asthmatic child because they restore the mucous membranes. These oils are found naturally in cod liver oil. It is interesting to note that in the 1940s children were given cod liver oil daily to help prevent chest infections and enhance nutrition. Cod liver oil is still a very good supplement. It can be taken in liquid or tablet form. Follow the instructions on the bottle depending on the age of your child.

- Ask your naturopath or herbalist for a tonic with equal parts of the following herbs: wild cherry bark (helps fight a nasty cough), echinacea (helps the immune system and upper respiratory tract), liquorice (soothes inflammation), chamomile (soothes and relaxes muscles), mullein (helps mucous to be coughed up), Cats claw (stimulates the immune system to fight viral infection) and elecampane (helps stop mucous production). For children aged over five years, give half to 1 teaspoon in half a glass of warm water or juice three times a day. The herbs are best mixed with sweet juice, or added honey if your child is fussy on taste.

- To help keep your child's fluid intake strong, and to clear congestion in the nose and chest, use a tea made from equal parts of organic chamomile, peppermint and spearmint. My Summer Delight tea (see page 128) contains these herbs with added calendula flowers, and it's a safe formula for children over the age of five.

# Asthma and antibiotics

We are all born with good and bad bowel flora, which play a role in breaking down food substances. With continual use of antibiotics, our natural bowel flora are depleted, which can lead to bloating, poor digestion and thrush. If your child is undergoing a course of antibiotics and suffers from stomach pain or cramps, it is vital not only to follow the asthma program already described, but also to include yoghurt with added acidophilus in their daily diet. It is also advisable to give acidophilus powder, half a teaspoon mixed with a little water, twice a day before meals. This will help regenerate natural bowel flora.

## ✱ Asthma and exercise

Exercise is very important for asthmatic children but it can trigger an attack. It is therefore vital to talk to your doctor in order to create a safe exercise program for your child. A lung capacity test can be performed to assess if your child needs salbutamol (Ventolin), or some other form of assistance, to open their lungs and reduce aggravation. Immunity-enhancing herbs and vitamins can still be taken and do not interfere with these preventative drugs.

Swimming is a very suitable exercise because it opens the lungs and helps correct and regulate breathing. Gym work, ballet dancing, yoga, running, basketball and all forms of upper-body exercise are also safe and excellent options. Make sure you and your child choose sports that they enjoy and are happy to play regularly.

## CASE STUDY

A woman brought her five-year-old daughter, Sophie, to see me. Sophie had been diagnosed with asthma but was allergic to the drugs prescribed by her doctor.

I felt that Sophie was too young and frail to have blood taken for a food allergy test, so I asked her mother to work with me on a trial-food basis by eliminating dairy, wheat and any food colourings from Sophie's diet for eight weeks. We replaced the dairy with soy milk, used rye bread and stopped sweets and canned foods. Sophie appeared to be worse at the change of seasons, so to boost her immune response to airborne allergens I made a liquid herbal tonic of echinacea glycetract (50 per cent), thyme (10 per cent), peppermint (10 per cent), grindelia (a herb specific for children's asthma) (10 per cent), chamomile (10 per cent) and marshmallow (10 per cent). I also put Sophie on a liquid iron tonic to boost her natural haemoglobin for oxygen intake (she did not like red meat).

Three weeks later Sophie returned without a wheeze, with colour in her face and a lot happier. She said she felt much better on the medicine. So I continued this treatment for another two months.

During the summer I allowed Sophie to eat high-allergy foods once a week. When the next winter months came I again put her on a stricter program with both tonics and extra vitamin C powder (200 mg per day taken in juice).

I noticed that when Sophie had a slight wheeze she had generally been playing in the cold air late in the afternoons. In these cases, I gave her an extra dose of medicine.

Sophie is now twelve years old and has completely grown out of asthma, is happy and is aware that if she eats high-allergy foods or gets run down at school she develops tightness in the chest. She swims and plays netball, which also assists her breathing.

# 3
# Earaches and tonsillitis

Earaches and tonsillitis do not always occur concurrently but they can aggravate each other.

If tonsillitis becomes chronic, infection can quickly spread in the upper respiratory areas such as ears and nose. In fact, infection can begin in the nose or sinus area and then travel to the tonsil area, through the Eustachian tube (the tube going from the sinuses to the ears) and into the ear drum.

During tonsillitis or a sinus attack, a child will also often have blocked ears; a doctor can check infection in these areas. Sometimes it is purely a mucous build-up or, if your child continues to complain about their hearing or you notice them not hearing you, it may be a wax build-up in the ears, and your doctor can clear this. Do not use anything in the ears unless prescribed.

# ✼ Earaches

Earaches can be a nasty and very painful addition to a cold, and can often occur when children spend time out in the chilly winter air. An earache can be a symptom of infection, especially if your child frequently suffers from throat infections. Bacteria can travel through the sinus passages to the ears and throat very rapidly, and if the infection is not attended to quickly, the eardrum can burst.

If your child's symptoms include a slight hearing problem or a continual runny nose, they may be suffering from glue ear, which is caused by excess mucous in the nasal cavities and leads to a wax build-up in the ears. Mucous build-up can be caused by genetic predisposition, allergies, colds or even continual bouts of tonsillitis, and can be aggravated by swollen tonsils and adenoids (see the box on page 41). In severe cases of glue ear, grommets are placed in the ears to allow them to properly drain the mucous, but this must be done by a doctor.

# Treatment

Natural medicine can be a useful first resort for treating earaches, infections and glue ear, but if your child does not rapidly improve, you must consult a specialist. (Children suffering from glue ear often need this entire treatment consistently for four to six months. You can use the treatment when grommets are in place, but reduce the frequency to once a day.)

Heat is lost very quickly through the top of the head, and cold winds and seasonal changes often bring on infections and earaches in children. So, the best defence against earaches and infections is to always ensure your child covers their ears and head with a warm hat during winter and in the cold evening air.

When dealing with earaches, it is important to boost your child's immunity (see also treatment recommendations on pages 11–13), because a strong immune system is sometimes all a child needs to arrest further development of infection. If your child's earache is not advanced and they are not in severe pain (your child may complain of slight pain but is not in any distress; is possibly lethargic, off-colour or has a runny nose), use the following treatment.

# earaches and tonsillitis

- Include onions in your child's daily diet, as well as spicy food such as ginger and chilli (if your child will eat them).

- Peppermint tea daily is a must because the natural menthol ingredient of peppermint assists in clearing the mucous. Give your child 1 cup with honey three times a day.

- A powder form of vitamin C with bioflavonoids is vital for your child's immune system and will help drain excess mucous. For children aged five to eight, give half a teaspoon three times a day; for children aged eight to twelve, give 1 teaspoon twice daily.

- Include garlic in your child's diet. Garlic contains an ingredient called allicin, which helps as a natural antibiotic. Give 1 garlic oil capsule two to three times a day to help kill bacteria.

- A herbal tonic is essential. Your herbalist or naturopath can make the following tonic for you: echinacea glycetract (50 per cent), thyme (10 per cent), peppermint (10 per cent), mullein (10 per cent), albizia (10 per cent) and marshmallow (10 per cent). For children aged five to seven, give half a teaspoon three times a day; for children aged eight to twelve, give three-quarters of a teaspoon three times a day.

- Teach your child to use a Vicks inhaler or spray at night if they are breathing poorly.

- Warm chamomile tea helps inflammation and is very comforting. Serve with honey.

- Switch a vaporiser – available at pharmacies – on in your child's room an hour before they go to bed, to clear the air and help your child breathe freely during the night. You can also add a few drops of eucalyptus or peppermint oil.

> **Adenoids**
>
> Adenoids sit at the back of the nose above the roof of the mouth. They are a spongy tissue that acts similarly to tonsils, as a line of defence against bacteria and viruses. A child's adenoids generally shrink in size after the age of three. If a child finds difficulty breathing, or their breathing (while normal) is noisy and rattly during the day, and the child has continual sore throats and swollen glands, adenoids need to be treated.

# Dos and don'ts

**Do**: Explain the big picture to your child so they understand why they are undergoing this treatment on a regular basis and for such a long time.

**Do**: Keep dairy products including ice-cream and cheese to a minimum, because they can encourage mucous formation in many children. As an alternative to dairy, use goat's, soy or UHT milk.

**Don't**: Place any object in your child's ears in an attempt to clear blockages or ear wax. If this is necessary it must be done by a doctor.

**Don't**: Put any type of oil in your child's ears, because it can be very dangerous. Only use prescribed drops from your doctor.

## ✳ Tonsillitis

The tonsils are two small glands in the back of the throat. They are the body's first line of defence against bacterial and viral infections. They also help stop any infections going through to the sinus area and bronchial tubes.

When infected, the tonsils swell and develop small white dots that become infected, causing soreness of the throat, lethargy, irritability, poor breathing, snoring due to blocked passageways, bad breath due to bacteria, and sometimes fever.

Most parents have some understanding of the swollen-tonsil syndrome and the symptoms that go with this nasty complaint. In the past, particularly the 1960s–80s, children suffering from tonsillitis were often sent straight to the hospital to have their tonsils removed, but now many doctors are very reluctant to remove tonsils except in very severe cases. General treatment by the medical profession these days is short- or long-term antibiotics.

Continual tonsillitis attacks can cause problems for children when they begin school, because tonsillitis can cause the oxygen supply to the brain to be reduced; the infection can irritate the ears and lower hearing, which can lead to learning difficulties. Children can also often lose their appetite, hence supplementation is vital.

Each tonsillitis case must be considered individually, but I have set out the following preventative program to assist the cases that do not need surgery. The program can prevent surgery in some cases, but the medicine needs to be used very quickly and frequently at the beginning of an attack in order to reduce the bacterial inflammation.

If you follow this program and your child is not better within 24 to 48 hours, you should see your doctor; your child will need to take a short course of antibiotics. It is important to note that natural herbs can be given simultaneously with the antibiotics unless your child has a very sensitive stomach; in these cases, you may use the herbs after the round of antibiotics has been completed, in order to boost your child's immune system.

Children who have only the occasional tonsillitis attack usually respond well to natural medicine, especially if they continue to take their tonics (see treatment below) throughout winter. In chronic cases you may need to run an antibiotic (see your doctor) alongside natural medicine.

If your child suffers from constant symptoms and infections from tonsillitis, I recommend you see a specialist for advice. In some exceptional cases, your child's tonsils and possibly their adenoids will have to be removed.

# Treatment

- Your child will not be able to eat or chew whole foods, so give plenty of fluids. Soups, soft cooked vegetables and fruits are excellent at this time.

- Honey is an antibacterial food, which most children enjoy. Children can eat honey from a spoon three to four times a day or chew on some pure honeycomb. I also recommend a gargle of warm water containing half a teaspoon of echinacea, a pinch of salt and half a teaspoon of honey.

- Ask your naturopath or herbalist for a tonic made with: echinacea (echinacea glycetract for children aged five to seven) (40 per cent), thyme (10 per cent), chamomile (10 per cent), baptisa (10 per cent), sage (10 per cent), myrrh (10 per cent) and peppermint (10 per cent). For children aged between two and five, give 10–20 drops in milk or juice four times a day. For children aged over five, give half a teaspoon in juice every 4 hours. When your child improves, use three times a day for three weeks. Then follow the section on boosting the immune system (see pages 11–13).

- Ask your health food store for a quality mix of vitamin C powder with bioflavonoids. Use half a teaspoon in juice three times a day.

## CASE STUDY

A nine-year-old boy, Mathew, came to visit me with his parents, who were exasperated because their son had been prescribed five sets of antibiotics during winter for tonsillitis. After examination, I noticed that Mathew's tonsils were very large for his age and he tended to speak and breathe in a muffled way. For the last three years Mathew had suffered this debilitating problem and doctors felt he was not a candidate for the removal of these glands.

To treat Mathew, I chose to use traditional herbs that focus on the upper respiratory tract and have a profound effect on stubborn causes of tonsillitis. I made a tonic of equal parts of *baptisia* (a native American herb), *echinacea angustofolia*, mullein and red raspberry leaf; I gave Mathew 1 teaspoon mixed in juice three times a day. I also gave him 100 mg of vitamin C three times a day and 1 garlic tablet three times a day. I asked Mathew to gargle with half a teaspoon of salt and 2 ml of myrrh in warm water twice a day.

As an added problem, Mathew tended to have bouts of diarrhoea due to long-term use of antibiotics. He did not like yoghurt, so we gave him half a teaspoon of acidophilus powder in half a glass of water twice a day before food.

Mathew came back after a month. He was feeling much better, had more energy and only a slightly swollen tonsil on one side.

Mathew kept on his medicine for four months. Following this, I stopped the tonic and acidophilus but asked him to continue with vitamin C for another two months.

Six months later Mathew had a mild attack and we repeated this treatment for six weeks.

Mathew is now eleven and has an occasional attack, which he manages to control with my herbs and vitamins. He is happier, healthier and has not had an antibiotic for the last two years.

# 4
# The brain

From the embryo through to childhood and adulthood, the brain changes and develops. It is the most remarkable organ and one of the least understood in the body.

> **Brain development**
>
> Although this book does not cover pregnancy and infancy, I would like to highlight some things a mother can do to optimise brain development in her child. It is essential to note that a pregnant woman should not smoke during her forty weeks' gestation. Cadmium in cigarettes can have a detrimental effect on an embryo, restricting oxygen flow to cell tissue and leading to a lower birth weight.
>
> For women who are trying to fall pregnant, I recommend a supplement of folic acid, to be continued throughout pregnancy. This supplement

> is believed to prevent spina bifida in children. It is believed that folic acid, a naturally occurring B vitamin found in green leafy vegetables and meats, is essential for the neurological functioning of many brain elements, although research is ongoing. Folic acid (folate) lowers homoscyteine levels in adults; high homoscyteine levels have been found to increase the tendency for cardiovascular disease and Alzheimer's disease, particularly in men.
>
> I also recommend a multivitamin for all women during pregnancy, even those with a healthy, balanced diet, because multivitamins are advantageous to the healthy growth of the embryo in the womb.

# Concentration

Concentration levels vary radically in children. At the extreme end, we know of problems such as hyperactivity, learning difficulties and Attention Deficit Hyperactivity Disorder (ADHD); at the other end of the scale is the seemingly simple case of needing to improve a child's concentration to allow them to approach school and life with confidence. I will discuss the extreme cases later in this chapter (see pages 54–67), but the more straightforward cases can be dealt with through regular supplements of vitamins and herbs. I have created the following program to help improve your child's concentration.

## Treatment

- Fresh foods are always the best foods for concentration, so avoid additives and colourings in your child's diet.

- Give your child small meals frequently. This prevents sugar highs and lows, which tend to make a child irritable and nervy, which in turn interferes with concentration.

- Your child should always eat breakfast. Include a carbohydrate and a protein, such as cereal with a boiled egg and toast, an omelette, tuna or sardines on toast, baked beans on toast, or even soup. Always incorporate fresh fruit or juice before or after protein, or pour it over cereal. Fruit clears the bowel of waste and gives the brain the antioxidant vitamin C, which combats free radical damage throughout the body, including the brain.

- Omega 3 essential fatty acids are vital for the healthy development of your child's neurological processes. These fatty acids have a profound effect on building healthy myelin sheaths around nerve tissue, and also assist the development of neurological pathways in the early stages of a child's life. These fatty acids are found in cod liver oils (which you can buy in health food stores) and in deep-sea fish. Supplementation can be given as young as twelve months, or when a child begins solids (see dosages on page 53). I believe that a child needs these supplements until the age of twelve. I have seen remarkable toning effects on the nervousness of hyperactive children in particular.

### Bacopa

*Bacopa monniera*, also known by its Sanskrit name, Brahmi, is found in damp and marshy areas of India. It has been used as a nerve tonic in the traditional Ayurvedic system, and recent studies have shown that the active substances, saponins Bacoside A & B, improve concentration, reduce anxiety and, in some cases, insomnia. Bacopa has often been referred to as a 'brain tonic' and is becoming highly respected in the treatment of nervous exhaustion in children (and adults).

# Supplements

- I always recommend a multivitamin with all the range of Bs (include $B_3$, $B_1$, $B_5$, $B_6$, $B_{12}$ and folate), because this vitamin assists concentration and is water soluble, and therefore has no sudden side effects. This multivitamin is essential when children are developing rapidly, especially around the age of eight to twelve, when schoolwork becomes more arduous.

- Omega 3 and 6 oils are essential. Omega 3 oils are found in fish oils, and omega 6 oils are found in vegetable oil, particularly flaxseed; you can buy a combination oil. For children aged five and over, give 1 teaspoon of each twice daily.

- Herbs such as bacopa and ginkgo (which assists circulation to the brain for short-term memory) can be given to children five years or older, but only in drop dosage; give 10 drops once a day after food as a combination tonic.

> ### Sleep is essential
>
> Sleep is essential for a child's concentration, and also if a child is bedwetting or having emotional problems. For restless sleepers, herbs can help. Try a short course of equal parts of chamomile and passionflower (use the tincture from a health food store or your naturopath) mixed into warm milk or water, half an hour before your child goes to bed: for children aged four to five, give 10 drops; add another

> 10 drops for each year of age after that.
>
> In addition to supplements, there are some routines you can put in place to help your child sleep. Make sure your child winds down an hour before bed and spends some time doing something quiet and calming, such as reading. Television stimulates the brain wavelengths and can keep a child's brain active for hours, so set strict rules for watching television, and ban violent or disturbing shows.

# ✲ Attention Deficit Hyperactivity Disorder (ADHD)

Attention Deficit Disorder (or syndrome), often referred to as ADD, or, when extra hyperactivity is present, Attention Deficit Hyperactivity Disorder (ADHD), is said to effect 2–9 per cent of school-age children, predominantly boys.

I will refer to both of these as ADHD because this is the most common behavioural disorder in childhood. By definition ADHD is characterised by inattention and being easily distracted, hyperactivity and impulsiveness; in most cases there is a combination of these. Symptoms include temper tantrums, an inability to cope with tasks, mood swings, disorganisation, antisocial behaviour and an inability to cope with stress. Research into ADHD is in its infancy and at this stage diagnosis is empirical, with no objective confirmations available from a blood test or a laboratory. If you suspect that your child is suffering from ADHD, consult your doctor for confirmation.

Drug medication currently on the market does not suit every child. Natural medicine has a lot to offer in terms of building a child's nervous system, and a naturopath can help teach parents and children about ways to avoid aggravating the situation. Special counsellors for this disorder can also be very helpful. (Your doctor can refer you to an appropriate counsellor.)

Various factors are believed to influence a child's susceptibility to ADHD. Genetics can play a role, as can exposure to heavy metals and pollutants, which disturb the neurological balance of the brain receptors. Scientists are trying to find evidence to link ADHD with prenatal stress; factors such as smoking, nutrition, socioeconomic status, family trauma and abusive parental behaviour can all possibly play a role.

Food additives, food allergies and sensitivity to environmental chemicals, moulds and fungi can play a major role in ADHD. In particular, many hyperactive children are sensitive to artificial colourings, flavours, preservatives and sometimes salicylates.

> ### Salicylates
>
> Salicylates are found in tomatoes, beans, capsicums, olives, most fruits (except bananas and peeled pears), almonds, peanuts and some seasonings (except garlic, parsley and chives). If your child is allergic to aspirin (part of the same family), they may also be allergic to foods containing salicylates. Keep this in mind when using the diet on pages 60–3.

The current medical treatment for ADHD is a drug called Ritalin (methylphenidate), which improves dopamine levels in the brain, which in turn improves the length of time a child can focus their attention. This drug has a considerable calming effect on ADHD children. One of the concerns about Ritalin is that some children have reported that the drug makes them feel extremely calm and not like their normal self; but the main concern is that it may suppress growth in children. Research is continuing in this area.

From a naturopathic point of view and in my experience, symptoms of ADHD can be dramatically reduced by cutting out food additives and colouring, minimising allergic reactions to foods and surroundings, and introducing herbs and vitamins. Each case is of course individual, but I strongly advocate trying these alternatives in diet and natural remedies before resorting to Ritalin. The following program can help reduce ADHD symptoms in children.

# Treatment

- Remove wheat, corn, milk, eggs, chocolate, oranges and citrus fruit from your child's diet. Include fresh fruits and vegetables, rice and other non-wheat/corn grains daily; also include chemical-free proteins such as fresh fish, chicken, red meats and legumes.

- For fluid intake, serve only fresh water, herbal teas, diluted fresh fruit juices and soups.

- Keep your child away from industrial chemicals such as PCBs, dioxins, chlorobenzenes, phenols and related chemicals, which have been found to increase the likelihood and severity of ADHD. These chemicals can be found in industrial areas or areas on main highways with petrol fumes.

- When considering how to improve your child's diet if they suffer from ADHD, poor concentration or behavioural issues, remember that as a parent you control the food buying in the home. The first step is to throw out all sweets, lollies, flavoured drinks such as Coke, Fanta and cordial, packet cake mixes and any tinned food that contains food colourings.

- Set aside time each week, preferably twice a week, to shop for the following:
  - fresh fruit and vegetables
  - proteins such as red meat, chicken and fish (you can

freeze these proteins and defrost them during the week as needed)
- legumes such as split peas, lima beans and adzuki beans (they are dried, so soak them overnight before cooking), which can be added to vegetables and soups
- eggs (but only if your child is not allergic)
- tinned salmon and tuna (with no additives)
- colouring-free bread that is based on rice flour or rye flour without yeast (ask your local health food store for a bread that is popular with children)
- try grains such as brown rice and buckwheat, and wheat-free pasta.

When you have the basics, make a rough outline of what you will cook for the three meals each day; include the rest of your family, who can eat in a similar fashion. In my clinical work I have found that the problem is often not so much in eliminating certain foods and additives from a child's diet, but rather how to bring healthier foods – foods they will enjoy – into their regular life. See the following pages for diet suggestions, and for further menus and recipes, see chapter 10.

# Diet to minimise the effects of ADHD, poor concentration and behavioural issues

## Breakfast

Remember, this meal is essential for a child struggling with any form of ADHD. Choose one of the following options.

- One to two boiled eggs with two slices of toast (special rye-based bread).

- Rice porridge with 1–2 teaspoons of ground almonds sprinkled on top.

- A tin of sardines, or tuna, salmon or mackerel on toast with a little tomato.

- Boiled brown rice mixed with vegetables (from the previous night's dinner), which can be made into a pan-fried pancake (you can add a raw egg to bind the ingredients together).

- An Asian-style soup with minimal spice.

## Snacks

- Sugarless dried fruit bars.

- A toasted or plain sandwich filled with chicken, red meat, cheese or salad.

- Fruit (fresh or stewed).

- Nuts (if your child is not allergic).

- Dried cracker biscuits with cheese, tuna or nut paste.

## Lunch

- A sandwich (made with rice-based bread), filled with a protein that your child enjoys and that does not go soggy, such as chicken, beef, egg, ham (no additives) or legumes (if mashed into a paste, such as chickpeas). Serve the sandwich with potato salad or some raw vegetable sticks such as carrot, celery or capsicum.

- A brown rice salad mixed with a protein and vegetables that don't go soggy, such as carrots, celery or zucchini.

- Rice or pasta salad with a protein and your child's favourite vegetables.

- If allowed at school, a hot thermos of vegetable and chicken soup, served with rice-based bread.

Note: Always include a treat such as a boiled lolly (without additives), a handful of organic dried fruit or a rice-flour biscuit with honey.

## Dinner

Always give your child a protein with three steamed or stir-fried vegetables of three different colours.

- Roast chicken or other meat, with vegetables.

- Casseroles with legumes, chicken, vegetables, served on brown rice or buckwheat.

- Stir-fried vegetables, chicken or meat served with pasta, buckwheat or rice.

- Thick legume and vegetable soup, served with toast and salad.

- Grilled fish, served with vegetables and salad.

> **Schisandra (*Schisandra chinensis*)**
>
> In the Chinese medical system, schisandra is regarded as one of the great antioxidant herbs. It has an amazing ability to detoxify the liver and to improve mental performance, and also physical performance and endurance. Schisandra has also been used successfully in chronic coughs and asthma.

# Supplements

- Vitamin B complex is essential in the treatment of ADHD. For children aged six or above, give 1 tablet daily – you can use a vitamin crusher and mix the tablet into yoghurt or other food. For children whose symptoms are very severe, give another B complex after lunch to assist in countering concentration falls and mood swings in the afternoon.

- ADHD children are significantly lower in essential fatty acids, especially omegas 3 and 6. Buy a good-quality liquid from your health food store; give 1 teaspoon twice daily.

- *Bacopa monniera* is an Indian herb that helps nervous exhaustion and stress, and can enhance mental performance (see the box on page 52). I recommend 1 tablet daily for children over six years old. The antioxidant schisandra is also wonderful: give 2 ml in water once daily. You can also mix bacopa and schisandra together in a tonic; give 20 drops twice a day. For children aged over eight, you can increase the dosage to three-quarters of a teaspoon, especially during times of mental and physical stress.

- Particular attention should be paid to the liver of a child with ADHD, because the liver is the organ that is sensitive to internal and external toxins. I recommend some form of liver detoxification and protection, such as a tonic made with equal parts of dandelion root, St Mary's thistle, rosemary and marshmallow (the latter gives a pleasant flavour). For children aged over six, give half a teaspoon once or twice a day. The healthy diet in chapter 10 is a natural detox for children. Note that a child should never detox with severe diets. I recommend children detoxing on soups and juices, only over the age of twelve, and only for two days.

- Your doctor or naturopath can test your child to see if they have been exposed to heavy metals, which can cause or aggravate ADHD. To assist the body to cleanse heavy-metal pollution, use dandelion root and St Mary's thistle with a vitamin B complex of 25–50 mg of the B spectrum taken once a day. Garlic also helps reduce harmful cadmium and mercury in the body; for children aged six or over, include 1 garlic tablet in the diet regularly.

- Chamomile tea is very calming. Give your child organic loose-leaf chamomile tea twice a day, especially before bed. The leaves can also be mixed (50/50) with a warm glass of soy or rice milk.

- Digestion problems and stomach cramps can be soothed by my Apres tea mixture (see page 127) – chamomile, fennel, aniseed and peppermint. This tea also aids the nervous system, and I particularly recommend it for children with colicky symptoms.

- A tablet of magnesium, calcium, manganese and zinc is very calming to the nervous system and helps hyperactive children sleep and grow, especially if they are not taking dairy products. Check with your naturopath for a suitable dose for your child.

### ADHD and psychological history

A definite link has been found between the nature of maternal care and a child's brain and psychological development. The link is especially marked in relation to the development of a child's behavioural patterns. For example, a child with a stressed mother may well become stressed. When a child perceives stress, they release stress hormones – glucocorticoids and catecholamines. Children of depressed parents commonly inherit not only a predisposition for depression but very often endure the compromised parental care of a depressed parent.

# 5
# The anxious child

Although anxiety is classed as a symptom and not a disease, children (just like adults) show signs of anxiety at different times. Anxiety in children can relate to stress, school, the home environment, peer pressures, achievements and growth spurts during which their body realigns and often requires a nutritional boost.

Herbal medicine has a long history in the treatment of nerves and anxiety. Tonics, nervines and restorative herbs have been used over hundreds of years in teas, liquid extracts and essential oils to assist the symptoms of anxiety and restlessness. Unfortunately, it is unlikely that a general doctor would treat these symptoms in children, because pharmaceutical drugs would not address the issues. In fact, these children respond brilliantly to an examination of lifestyles and diet – what we refer to as a holistic overview where a naturopath or herbalist can diagnose and treat anxiety symptoms with calming, safe herbs and simultaneously an added vitamin to see the child through this time.

# Anxiety

Children are continually learning new skills to cope with anxiety and pressures from their environment, but unfortunately some children do not cope well. If your child is prone to anxiety, they need lots of general rest and quality sleep, healthier foods and herbal tonics to assist and build a healthy nervous system. Rest assured (and reassure your child) that there is nothing wrong with this. We are all built differently, and children tend to show visible signs of needing this extra care during the tender developmental years of five to twelve.

The anxious child may not necessarily be hyperactive, suffer from ADHD (see the section on ADHD on pages 54–7) or have learning difficulties. The anxious child often shows symptoms such as sleeplessness, biting nails, withdrawing from discussing problems, sudden outbursts of temper or mood swings, worrying over small things, weepiness, shyness and timidity.

A child can often become anxious following a traumatic experience such as a car accident, parents' separation, or physical or mental abuse from family, siblings or peers.

## Treatment

- It is important to provide your child with a stable home environment. Keep any disagreements well beyond earshot of your child, and create a feeling of security when talking through any issues. Observe your child in different circumstances, to ascertain whether something specific is troubling them. Watch how your child relates to each member of your family or peer group.

- Anxious children often show their anxiety in their stomach. They can complain of stomach-aches and become quite irritable after eating certain foods. Record what upsets their stomach and make the child aware of the problem. If your child has a stomach-ache, a cup of peppermint tea (with some honey and chamomile to taste) is an excellent carminative.

- Make sure your child's nutritional needs are well covered with three healthy meals a day. If your child is not eating, a little care is needed for a while until they regain their appetite. Tempt them with a favourite (but healthy) meal, such as chicken and vegetable soup or spaghetti bolognaise. Work with foods that are healthy and your child enjoys, and include these in fun foods such as rissoles, pancakes or nutritional milkshakes.

- Cut back on all colourings in foods. Stop or minimise sugar treats, because sugar leaches from the body precious vitamins that feed your child's nervous system.

> ### Calcium
> Calcium is essential for every growing child, and it is particularly important for the anxious child because calcium is a calming mineral. Incorporate yoghurt and white cheese into your child's diet, and give two glasses of milk each day (try goat's milk if your child is allergic to cow's milk). A warm milk before bed with added passionflower or chamomile tea is very calming to an anxious child.

- If your child is anxious and a poor eater, I recommend a liquid iron tonic: 1 teaspoon twice a day until improvement.

- Mix half a teaspoon of magnesium powder with calcium in milk or water after dinner. Children cope so much better at exam time if they have added minerals.

- A herbal tea made from organic chamomile, vervain and oat straws is wonderful on a daily basis to relax your child and build a healthy nervous system.

- To help your child relax and sleep peacefully, add 6 drops of lavender and 6 drops of chamomile essential oil to a warm bath before bed.

- St John's wort (*Hypericum*) assists children aged under twelve with mild depression and anxiety. Give 25–30 drops in juice or water twice a day until improvement.

- Passionflower is an excellent herb for children who suffer nervous headaches or are very irritable. Passionflower herb has been used in traditional Western herbal medicine for the last 100 years, especially for insomnia and nervous irritability. For children aged five to twelve, give 10 drops once or twice a day. To assist sleep, give 20 drops in a glass of milk before bed.

> ### Herbal tonics
>
> It is very safe to give your child herbal tonics for six to twelve months. A naturopath can make these tonics for you and clarify the appropriate dose for your child, and can then adjust the herbs as your child improves. The herbs used in these tonics are safe and effective. The only side effect your child may experience is a feeling of nausea if they take the tonic on an empty stomach. Like vitamins, tonics need food or milk to assist their absorption.

# Dos and don'ts

**Do**: Be patient with your anxious child. They are highly sensitive and often react acutely to stress.

**Do**: Nurture with love and kindness. Encourage your child to talk about anything that is worrying them. Don't be upset if they feel more comfortable opening up to a good friend or another family member than to you.

**Do**: Use honey instead of white sugar to sweeten foods.

**Do**: Remember that it is very important to build your child's nervous system – it is as important as building the respiratory and immune systems.

**Don't**: Force your child to eat something they do not like. Work with any healthy foods they like, and serve these foods for breakfast, lunch and dinner until your child is ready to try something new. After eating a good meal, you can reward your child with a healthy dessert such as stewed fruit and a small spoonful of (preservative-free) ice-cream, or some carob or cornflake-and-honey crackles.

# Restlessness

Put simply, restlessness in children can be just part of growing up. Children have much to take on as they grow and learn about the world. We sometimes forget that children have many factors in their lives that can cause stress, and they do not always have the ability or vocabulary to communicate the significance of the stress they feel to their parents or peers. As such, it is vitally important that we take the time to properly observe the 'restless child' when deciding on treatment.

Common symptoms of restlessness include sleeplessness, unusual alertness before bedtime, mood swings, constipation, agitation, unusual fidgeting, constant swinging of the legs while seated, bursts of anger, nail-biting and waking through the night (this can include bedwetting).

# Treatment

Herbal medicine is a safe and effective method of treating this problem, and it has a very long history of restoring the nervous system to its equilibrium.

- Diet can play a significant role in relieving tension and restlessness. If your child is suffering from restlessness, it is important to follow the child's healthy diet outlined in chapter 10. Follow the diet for three months and keep a record of any foods that seem to cause bad-tempered behaviour in your child (usually within two to three hours after consumption); record your observations in a notebook over the three months. From this, you will be able to see if there are any foods that seem to set off mood swings; avoid those foods.

- If your child complains of being hungry between meals, give them healthy snacks, because it is possible they are going through a growth spurt and need protein and vegetables every three to four hours.

- Remove stimulants (including fizzy drinks and artificially coloured drinks and foods) at least four hours before your child goes to bed. Television and computer work should be finished at least three hours before bed.

- Observe your child's toileting habits and see if your child is constipated. If so, this can be treated with herbs and attention to diet (see the section on constipation in chapter 7, pages 98–102).

> **Chamomile (German *Matricaria recutita*)**
>
> The active ingredient in chamomile is its essential oil called chamazulene. Chamomile has been used since ancient times and is well known for its use in beverages, cosmetics, medicinal preparations and essential oils for perfumes.
>
> Chamomile is used specifically for calming treatments in nervous disorders and as a calmative for spasmolytic gastrointestinal tract; it makes a wonderful tea for colicky babies as young as six months. Chamomile is also widely known as a topical application for eczema and wound healing. For medicinal purposes always use organic chamomile.

# Supplements

- Chamomile, as a tea or a concentrated fluid extract. (The extract can be obtained from a herbalist.) Give 30–50 drops of the extract once a day, or 2–3 cups of the organic loose-leaf tea (add honey to taste) three times a day.

- Vervain, as a tea mixed with chamomile or a fluid extract, is a wonderful nervine tonic. If you are using it in extract form, give 30 drops in water or milk before bed. This herb can be used three times a day if your child is anxious.

- Magnesium is also a wonderful calmative. For children over the age of five, mix half a teaspoon of magnesium powder with calcium in milk or water at night.

- Rescue Remedy, a homoeopathic remedy made from the essence of flowers, is excellent for short-term use: 2 drops three times a day for two to three weeks.

- Ask your naturopath to make you a day tonic of equal parts of passionflower, vervain, chamomile and marshmallow: for children aged five to seven, give 10–20 drops three times a day until they improve; for children aged seven to twelve, give 20–40 drops. Mix this tonic in a glass of warm milk before bed, and it will help settle your child.

- To combat sleeplessness, ask your naturopath to make you

a tonic of equal parts of passionflower, vervain, scullcap and oats: for children aged five to seven, give 30 drops in warm water 30 minutes before bed; for children aged seven to twelve, give 50 drops. This is a little stronger than the passionflower–vervain–chamomile–marshmallow tonic described in the previous point.

## CASE STUDY

A six-year-old boy, Peter, came to visit me with his parents because they were concerned about his poor appetite and restless behaviour in his first year of school. When Peter wanted to concentrate at school he was very centred and socialised well with the other children. He did not seem to catch colds easily and was generally a happy child. However, when evenings came he refused to settle to bed, and when he finally did sleep he woke several times through the night.

I prescribed the passionflower–vervain–chamomile– marshmallow tonic (described in point five) to build his nervous system and ease growing pains (see section on growing pains on pages 83–5), which I believed could be causing his restlessness. I prescribed half a teaspoon three times a day, and an extra dose mixed in water in the middle of the night if he woke. I also prescribed a crushed tablet of calcium magnesium (which also contained zinc, manganese and other minerals that are suitable for children in this age group). The crushed tablet was placed in yoghurt in the evening. I asked Peter's parents to give him no sugar, including fruits, juices and ice-cream, after 5 p.m.

After three weeks Peter had improved by 50 per cent. He was going to bed earlier and was sleeping more soundly and consistently. He was still a little anxious through the day, so I asked his parents to increase the tonic dose to 1 teaspoon three times a day for the next six weeks.

I did not see Peter for three months but his parents kept him on the tonic for this time. On returning to see me, he was a much happier child – he was calmer and seemed easier to talk to. Peter now only takes the tonic when he feels he needs it to help him through a difficult time. Children often surprise me by how much they know; they will often ask their parents for their prescribed tonics because they 'feel much better on them'.

### Restless boys

Sometimes boys aged eight to twelve can go through a difficult patch. They can have problems with schoolwork, their peers and other children. If this is the case, it is important to establish that ADHD is not the issue, especially if your child is struggling with concentration (see the section on ADHD on pages 54–7).

Boys often burn the nutrients in the body at a faster rate than girls through sport and active play. In order to keep their energy levels high, I always recommend a vitamin B complex (a 20–40 mg tablet containing most of the Bs) for boys aged eight to twelve: 1 tablet daily. Give 1 calcium and magnesium tablet at night if they are growing rapidly and are restless or complaining of leg cramps.

# Dos and don'ts

**Do**: Read to your child before bed, to help them wind down.

**Do**: Turn off the television and computer three hours before bed.

**Do**: Initiate some quiet game-playing with your child an hour before their bedtime; try a card game, puzzle or their favourite board game.

**Do**: Provide a healthy breakfast each morning to give your child the fuel to concentrate at school.

**Do**: Provide healthy snacks in the afternoon when your child arrives home from school.

**Do**: Insist your child take their tonics, but do not call them medicines. Tell your child that the tonics will help build their body as sportspeople build theirs.

**Don't:** Give your child stimulants – such as caffeine or spicy food – before they go to bed.

**Don't**: Give your child food containing a lot of artificial colourings.

**Don't**: Ignore early warning signs such as unusual bad behaviour and unhappiness. Find out what the problem is.

**Don't**: Discount weather changes in relation to your child's restlessness; your child may have a virus or flu.

**Don't**: Allow your child to stay up late in the evenings, just to keep the peace. Observe the previous steps and find out why your child is not sleeping at night.

# Growing pains

This problem is often not obvious. Your child may find it difficult to explain their restlessness, especially during the night when they can experience cramps and aching legs.

In my clinical experience, I have often found that a child will tell me they have a pain or a sore body part (particularly the knees, calf muscles and ankles). Upon questioning the parent about the child's growth spurts, these symptoms often tie up with the child's rate of growth and increased appetite. 'My child eats me out of house and home' is often the joking comment from parents.

If your child is suffering from growing pains, you can usually address the problem by increasing their intake of protein, such as fish (tinned fish with bones, such as salmon and tuna, and sardines for added calcium), eggs (high in lecithin to assist brain function) and red meats (for iron content). Dairy products such as milkshakes, yoghurt and white cheese are good sources of calcium for bone development. If your child is allergic to dairy, buy a calcium–magnesium tablet or powder and give 1 tablet or half a teaspoon of the powder twice daily until their pains subside.

Children should be shown how to properly stretch before sport and after sitting at a computer or their homework desk. This not only helps circulation, but allows healthy ligament and cartilage around growing joints to work more efficiently. Sometimes if a child complains about an injury (from sport or in general), you can take them to see an osteopath, who can test whether your child has structural (skeletal–muscular) problems and also address problems such as flat feet, knocked knees, or having one leg shorter than the other. Addressing these issues at an early age can save long-term muscle and ligament pain as your child moves into adulthood.

# 6
# Skin conditions

Children often suffer distressing skin conditions that can be hereditary but can also appear during times of seasonal changes, stress, allergies, exposure to dust mites and overheating (caused by swimming in chlorinated heated swimming pools). Children are very self-conscious about their appearance, especially their skin, so it is important to remember that rashes, eczema and dermatitis all cause some form of emotional stress as well as physical discomfort in the child.

Mild skin conditions are often unsuccessfully treated by the medical profession, usually because varying elements – particularly environmental – are not adequately addressed. A health practitioner such as a naturopath can take a holistic approach to your child's skin problems and can work in conjunction with a general doctor.

Often a doctor will prescribe a low-dose cortisone-based cream for skin rashes and mild eczema, but natural medicine can play a significant role in lowering the severity of the attacks and controlling the frequency. On some occasions both can be used to gain a result, and a herbal-based ointment can then be introduced.

With all skin conditions in children, it is important to observe any change in condition and severity of attacks (a diet diary and a seasonal change diary can be kept). Therefore, if your child only suffers rashes during spring or autumn, they need to take preventative natural medicine as outlined below at least four weeks before and during that time.

# ✻ Eczema and other rashes

Rashes are more common in infants than in children aged five to twelve, but many children suffer varying degrees of eczema and/or sensitive skin due to the change of seasons, and through allergies to foods, fabrics and soaps.

Eczema can be a dry or wet, itchy and sometimes bleeding rash. Often eczema is hereditary, but it can be aggravated by allergy foods and environmental airborne allergens. The eczema rash is most often seen in crevices such as behind the knees or in the crease of the elbow, but it can also occur on the eyelids and in the crevices of the nose and ears.

Natural medicine can help you control these aggravating conditions in your child. Often these conditions run in families who show a genetic predisposition to some forms of allergies, especially asthma. Children often grow out of even severe cases of eczema, but in the meantime herbs, diet and omega oils are vital to the health of your child's skin. Most rashes respond well to the treatment I have outlined in this section.

# Preventative program

- Foods play a vital role in the prevention and treatment of eczema and other rashes. The following foods can aggravate eczema and should be eliminated from your child's diet for two months:
  - Spicy foods, which overheat the blood, especially chillies, curries and garlic. It is important to keep a food diary to see how these foods affect the skin; if they aggravate the skin within four hours of consumption, eliminate them for six weeks and try again.

## skin conditions

- All acidic foods and drinks (fresh or bottled), such as oranges, wheat products, peanuts, and refined sugars and colourings.
- Eggs – eliminate them from your child's diet for six weeks, then challenge their body by serving an egg every four days – if your child's skin becomes aggravated, eggs could be the cause.
- Dairy – some children are allergic to dairy, which can cause rashes. If you think this may be the case, ask your doctor to perform a food allergy test. If your child is allergic, try soy or goat's milk and yoghurt.

After two months without these foods, introduce each food, one at a time, every four days. If there is a flare-up of the skin following the reintroduction of a particular food, do not give this food to your child for another six weeks before trying again. Your child's skin will often improve radically when you eliminate the main allergy foods from your child's diet.

- For breakfast, serve rice porridge, cereal or a wheat-free toast spread with your child's favourite protein, such as soy paste, chickpea paste (hummus), almond paste or fish paste. For lunch and dinner, follow the listed restrictions and serve your child lots of cooked vegetables, which are very alkaline and reduce the body's heat. Give your child vegetable soups, mashed vegetables, roast vegetables and baked vegetables, accompanied by a protein such as fish or free-range chicken. All legumes are good, but introduce them to your child's diet slowly, through soups and casseroles, because many children are fussy about the taste and may reject legumes if they are served plain.

- Remove chemical soaps, detergents and dust mites (if practical, it is better to have no carpets) from your home, to decrease allergic reactions in your child. Dress your child in cottons or pure silk fabrics against the skin.

# Treatment for itchy skin

- Chickweed ointment is wonderful for the relief of itching. This cream has been used for centuries as an ointment for eczema.

- You can also try pinetarsol, which is readily available at pharmacies. Pinetarsol can be mixed into bath water and will temporarily relieve itching for children over the age of five (follow the directions for the dose). This product works very well but smells awful, so a few drops of lavender oil in the bath will mask the smell as well as help your child's skin.

- Sorbolene cream applied on a daily basis after showering or bathing assists dry skin – but remember, creams are temporary. While you treat your child internally with oils, herbs and vitamins, you must also cut out the allergens that cause the condition.

- Chamomile tea is an excellent calmative: give 1 cup a day either mixed in milk or sweetened with honey. Chamomile creams have a soothing effect on irritated skin and can be used frequently.

- Give 1 capsule of evening primrose oil daily. (If your child cannot swallow the capsule, open it and pour the oil on a spoon or mix it in half a teaspoon of honey for your child to take internally.)

> ### A remedy to relieve itchy skin
>
> Fill a muslin bag with 2–3 tablespoons of oats. Tie it over the bath tap so the water flows through the bag and the ingredients. Place your child in the lukewarm bath for 10 minutes before bed. This gives great relief for itchy skin and usually keeps the itching settled all night.

## Supplements

- Omega 3 and 6 oils are essential in repairing and preventing dry and itchy skin. Use a high-quality oil that does not contain added flavourings. These usually consist of fish oil and evening primrose oil with flaxseed oil. These oils are also essential for brain development and concentration, and I recommend every child take these supplements on a daily basis. Give 1 teaspoon twice daily.

## CASE STUDY

Eight-year-old Jessica suffered from eczema in summer; when she came to see me with her parents she had been suffering from this complaint for three years. Her parents had taken her to see their doctor, who performed a Rast skin test, but the test showed that she was not allergic to dairy, wheat or yeast. She ate a number of coloured jubes, which I reduced. She also told me she swam in the school swimming team, and that they trained in a chlorinated pool. I gave Jessica chickweed cream to soothe her itchy skin, and, slowly over two weeks, I reduced the steroid cream that her doctor had prescribed. I also gave her a tonic of equal parts of echinacea root blend, nettle and chamomile, prescribing 2.5 ml in water twice daily. I also gave Jessica 1 capsule of evening primrose oil daily.

Jessica came back to see me after six weeks of the treatment and showed considerable improvement; she reported that her eczema did not react as dramatically after swimming. We continued this program for ten months, and Jessica's improvement continued.

### Swimming and sunshine

Swimming in the ocean can dramatically relieve eczema, and mild sun on the skin in summer is a must. Vitamins A and D are produced by the body from the sun on the skin. These vitamins are essential to heal and cleanse eczema. (You will notice that it is often in the winter months that a child has breakouts of eczema and other rashes and needs extra oils and supplements.)

# 7
# The digestive system

Digestion is an important function in the overall health of a child. The digestive system has many parts that must all work in unison. Complicated enzymes are released from the salivary glands, the liver, gallbladder and pancreas to break down proteins, starch and fats. Inherited poor digestive systems in children as well as acquired sluggish digestive systems can cause major symptoms such as lethargy, wind, nausea, constipation, intolerance of fatty foods and bloated sensations often leading to stomach cramps.

Herbalists are very thorough in treating these symptoms because they believe that chronic diseases begin with poor digestive function, and good upper-digestive function is a prerequisite for a healthy digestive system. With children in particular, poor upper-digestive function can be a consequence of prolonged illnesses such as infections and anaemia.

I often see children who look pale and sickly, eat very little, tend to feel bloated and never seem to have the vital energetic force of the human physiology. These are all symptoms of a poor digestive system. Stimulation of gastric enzymes, examining food intolerances and checking the child's regular bowel habits are all important factors in the diagnosis of why the child is suffering from constipation, diarrhoea, stomach cramps or general debility.

Herbal medicine has a very important role to play in correcting digestion, because natural plants and foods contain enzymes, tannins, bitters, alkaloids and flavonoids, which all play a role in safely assisting normal digestion.

# Stomach upsets

Most children complain of stomach upsets on and off throughout childhood. The cause could be simply an overload of sugar, preservatives and additives from a birthday party. It could also be as simple as 24 to 48 hours of constipation. If the above are the reasons for the stomach upset, your child's body will repair itself as things pass out of their system.

General stomach upsets include abdominal pain, sometimes associated with constipation or diarrhoea. If the pain is severe, such as in the case of food poisoning, vomiting can occur. Children suffering from abdominal pain are generally irritable and lethargic, and can often have mood swings and exhibit poor behaviour.

There are many children who experience stomach-aches as a daily problem, and their parents often come to me beside themselves with worry. And rightly so, because Western medicine has very little to offer in this area, except to take a stool test to see if the child has worms or a bacteria in the faeces. Certainly, if symptoms persist and your child is in regular pain, it is worth a visit to your doctor to carry out these tests.

# Treatment

- If symptoms persist over a period of time (in some cases this can be as long as one to two years), the possibility of food allergies must be eliminated. Firstly, eliminate all food colourings and additives from your child's diet, and limit drinks to fresh nectar or 100 per cent fruit juices. Remove highly coloured lollies (especially red, orange and green), which can cause stomach upsets; if you must buy your child sweets as a treat, buy the ones that do not contain these colourings. Stick to this diet for three weeks and keep a diary of when your child complains of stomach pain; record the foods that seem to make your child feel unwell within three hours of eating. If pasta, wheat bread or eggs show in this diary, eliminate them and replace with rye or rice bread.

- Add fibre to your child's food, such as 1 teaspoon of psyllium husks on (oat or rice) porridge. Serve plenty of fresh, steamed vegetables in the evening meal. Only give your child the steamed vegetables they love, even if it is the same each evening. Also try a raw salad as a side dish to the evening meal.

- Chamomile and peppermint tea both ease stomach cramps, so serve as often as possible on a daily basis. A hot water bottle on the stomach area can also assist.

# Constipation

Children can become very irritable when changes in their bowel movements occur. Your child may feel uncomfortable discussing their bowel habits with you (this usually sets in around the age of six), so you may need to closely observe your child's toileting habits. If your child becomes very moody and spends a lot of time in the bathroom, they may be experiencing this problem.

Constipation can be caused at an early age by children trying to 'hang on' until they arrive home from school because they do not want to go to the toilet at school. Constipation can also be caused by food intolerances, particularly when children eat a lot of bread or have little fibre in their diet. On rare occasions children can inherit a particularly long bowel; in these cases, bowel motions take longer due to the length of the bowel. Your doctor can confirm this through an X-ray, if all other problems have been addressed.

# Treatment

- If your child is suffering from constipation, bring more fibre into their diet in the form of steamed, mashed or raw vegetables and fresh whole fruits; vegetable soups are a great after-school snack and are good for the bowel.

- Ensure your child is drinking water, herbal teas or a high-quality 100 per cent juice each day.

- Cut back on white-flour breads and pasta, and serve wholemeal breads that contain whole seeds. Children often dislike the taste of brown rice, so use a mixture of brown and white rice. Include raw foods such as celery, carrots, capsicum and lettuce.

- Make sure your child has a good, healthy breakfast in the mornings, particularly porridge or a cereal; you can include some psyllium husks sprinkled over the cereal, for added fibre.

- Ask your pharmacist to recommend the best fibre powder for your child.

- If your child is in pain, a hot-water bottle on the abdomen is a great comfort to spasmodic bowel muscles. Following a stomach-ache, warm chicken broth is comforting and easy to digest.

# Supplements

- Slow bowel motions can be assisted by acidophilus powder: give 1 teaspoon mixed into a little water once a day before dinner.

- Herbal tonics can clear the bowel and get rid of toxin build-up from food allergies and poor bowel habits. I use a wonderful tonic made from equal parts of dandelion root, liquorice, marshmallow and yellowdock; 3 ml in water twice daily.

- For children aged over six, give 1 teaspoon a day of aloe vera juice, especially if they have associated reflux with irregular bowel motions.

- Two to three prunes on top of a good-quality cereal with 1 teaspoon of psyllium husks is a great preventative for children's constipation.

- Whenever your child has been eating poorly, the following tea will assist in regular bowel motions and make your child feel better. Make a tea from 1 teaspoon each of roasted dandelion root, liquorice root and peppermint. Simmer in 1 litre of water for 15 minutes and sweeten with pure dark honey. Give your child 2–3 cups on the first day, and then give 1 cup daily until your child feels better.

# Diarrhoea

Diarrhoea can be very unpleasant for children. If diarrhoea does not respond to diet and natural medicine within 12 hours, you should consult your doctor, who can check if your child has an infection or other major problem.

Bouts of diarrhoea in a child are often related to diet, and often accompany a poor immune system. The child loses many nutrients and often has very poor assimilation of all food groups. That is why fresh and gently cooked food is essential. This assists the child's digestive system because it doesn't have to work so hard to break down nutrients in the food.

# Treatment

- Follow the treatment for stomach upsets (see pages 97–8).

- During bouts of diarrhoea, give your child honey mixed in warm water; this will help their sugar levels and keep up their energy. Lemonade is also helpful in stopping dehydration.

- Following a bout of diarrhoea, your child will need to eat every two to three hours. Mashed vegetables (but not tomatoes or eggplant) with boiled rice are ideal in the first few days. You can also serve boiled chicken, but fish and red meats are too heavy in the first few days after diarrhoea. If your child complains of feeling bloated after eating oat porridge, rice porridge is a delicious alternative (oats contain gluten but rice does not).

- Soups are an ideal after-school snack. Variety each day with vegetables and proteins is essential. Soups are also very alkaline and soothing, especially when served over white rice.

# Supplements

- Herbs and plants containing tannin and flavonoids are very useful to strengthen the wall of the bowel and are gentle for children. Try black tea, raspberry leaf tea and raw apples (apples contain pectin, a great natural cleanser for children that helps prevent diarrhoea). For children aged over five, black tea can be given two to three times a day (always serve one with the lowest caffeine level).

- Children also respond to a tea of meadowsweet, chamomile and peppermint, sweetened with honey to taste: give two to three times a day.

- Slippery elm bark, a powder that can be obtained from a health food store, acts as a soother and healer to your child's bowel wall. For children aged five and above, mix half a teaspoon with a little yoghurt and honey: give twice a day for two to four weeks.

- For children aged over five, half a teaspoon twice a day of magnesium powder will assist a lazy or loose bowel.

- For children aged five and above, I often recommend a natural liquid iron tonic for children, made from herbs and berries that are naturally high in iron and vitamin C. These tonics are available in different forms from health food stores. Only use this tonic after a diarrhoea attack and continue use for at least a month.

- Cinnamon is a delicious-tasting herb that assists digestion and an irritable bowel. Use freely to flavour your child's food, particularly cooked fruits and rice dishes.

- For children aged over eight, peppermint tea mixed with chamomile soothes the walls of the bowel and has a calmative effect to help your child to feel better. This tea is also useful as a gargle for bleeding gums or mouth ulcers.

> ### An old remedy for diarrhoea
>
> Boil half a cup of rice in 4 cups of water for 20 minutes. Strain off the water and allow it to cool. Give your child 1 teaspoon of the cooked rice, then wash down with sips of rice water. Keep your child sipping on the rice water for as long as possible until at least 1–2 cups have been consumed. This remedy can stop the worst of diarrhoea bouts.

## CASE STUDY

A couple brought their five-year-old daughter, Isabella, to see me as a last resort for her constipation and stomach cramps. She had seen doctors, but apart from a fibre called metamusil (which worsened her problems), nothing more was offered.

To try and obtain immediate relief (Isabella only moved her bowel once every three to four days), I gave her a tonic made from liquorice (40 per cent), dandelion root (40 per cent) and peppermint (20 per cent); 3 ml twice a day. I asked Isabella's parents to eliminate white bread from her diet and replace it with grainy bread. Isabella drank very little distilled water and herb tea, and only liked Fanta. Because of the orange 'flavour' in Fanta, I changed Isabella to two glasses of freshly squeezed orange juice daily. I also made sure she ate whole-wheat cereal each morning.

After three weeks Isabella and her parents returned. She was moving her bowel daily but still suffered some pain and bloating. I asked her parents to continue the treatment and added half a teaspoon of acidophilus powder in water twice a day. I also asked them to massage Isabella's bowel before bed, using a circular motion clockwise around the stomach region.

After another three weeks Isabella seemed much happier, less moody and was eager to continue the treatment.

I stopped the tonic three months later; now, after two years, Isabella has very few problems. Only if she becomes stressed or consumes a lot of bread or fizzy drinks does she need to take the tonic for one to two weeks.

# 8
# The four seasons

I am going to outline some basic principles for you to follow to maintain your child's health during all seasons and seasonal changes. I believe that the most common childhood ailments can be eliminated or reduced by following these preventative principles, which essentially build up a child's immune system to battle different threats at different times of the year. Careful preparation will also reduce the need for a 'quick fix', because your child is less likely to become ill.

> ### Juice
> Many juices and fruit drinks on the market are filled with added sugar. Unfortunately, this not only leads to extra kilojoules (weight) for a child but can have a tendency to burn up valuable vitamins while breaking down the overload of sugar. Try to freshly squeeze a juice once a day or give your child two to three pieces of whole fruit. When buying juice, look for:

- no added sugars
- no preservative
- added dietary fibre
- 100 per cent fruit juice.

## ✹ Summer

Always use a 30+ strength sunblock on your child's skin during the summer months. Train your child to wear a hat, long-sleeved shirt and zinc cream on their cheeks and nose when out in the sun for long periods of time.

Water is essential to ensure your child is properly hydrated. Make sure you also give your child plenty of freshly squeezed juices of the seasonal fruits. (You can also add fresh juice to water.) A banana a day will help alleviate dehydration by keeping your child's potassium and sodium levels balanced.

Children can lose sodium and electrolytes from their bodies when they sweat, so it is important to add a little sea salt to foods to counter these effects.

Summer is a good time to concentrate on establishing a very healthy diet. An apple a day assists bowel movements, because apples contain pectin, a great natural cleanser for children.

This is also a great time to introduce your child to different forms of fresh, deep-sea fish; serve them in salads and pasta dishes. You can also try light grains such as couscous; introduce them with your child's favourite vegetables and tomatoes, as well as fresh herbs such as mint or basil.

Light wholemeal pancakes are a delicious addition to your child's lunch box. Roll them up with salad and a protein such as chicken. Most children will be excited by this new type of sandwich.

I generally recommend giving a child a complete break from vitamins and herbal tonics during the summer months, because summer foods contain all the essential nutrients.

If you and your child are travelling to a cold country for our summer, prepare your child's immune system to face the change of weather three weeks prior to travelling (see chapter 1).

## ✳ Autumn

Autumn brings cooler months and a higher susceptibility to allergies in children. It is vital that children who have allergies to grasses and trees take a herbal supplement to build their immunity against these pollens.

If your child is prone to asthma, sinus or eczema, begin with a vitamin C with bioflavonoids; for children aged five to twelve, give 100–200 mg once a day. Also give 1 teaspoon of echinacea glycetract in liquid form once a day.

Air all winter clothes to eliminate dust mites and odour, which can cause allergy problems, especially for eczematous children. Children who are prone to skin rashes should wear cotton T-shirts or natural fibres under wool jackets or jumpers.

To prepare your child's skin for the drying effect of the change of seasons, use natural moisturising creams such as Sorbolene after bathing.

If your child does not have severe allergic problems but has a tendency to a lowered immunity when the weather changes (see chapter 1), a multivitamin tablet is essential.

Start changing your child's diet to include slightly heavier foods in the form of more carbohydrates and proteins that warm the body, such as (preferably brown) rice dishes, oat porridge and soups containing legumes and grains such as barley and split peas. If your child is not vegetarian, introduce some red meats twice a week, as well as free-range chicken and legumes. Often children 'go off' fish dishes during this time because fish is lighter and children need heavier proteins to sustain energy in the colder climate.

## ✱ Winter

Sudden drops in temperature and bitter wind changes can lower the body's heat energy very quickly and cause an imbalance in the natural life forces and the body's equilibrium. In traditional Chinese medicine and also in Western herbal medicine we take these elements very seriously. We make sure that we adjust our general living patterns and diets accordingly, with added herbs and supplements, and different seasonal foods. This approach also applies to our children. Always keep your child warm in the chest, head and kidney areas with a warm jacket and/or scarf and hat – these areas are where most body heat is lost.

As winter sets in, your child will naturally eat more foods to maintain body warmth. It is imperative that your child has a big – and preferably hot – breakfast in winter, for the prevention of coughs, colds and flus. Introduce your child to porridge, because oats raise body temperature; ground nuts on top of the porridge will give your child valuable protein in the morning before school. Other suitable breakfasts include hot eggs or an omelette, and wholemeal toast with a legume such as baked beans.

Make sure you guide your child towards healthy – preferably hot – snacks (see the snacks section, pages 142–5). Bananas and nuts with some dried fruits make great morning tea (recess) snacks; after school, try toasted sandwiches, hot vegetable soups and hot pasta and noodle dishes. Remember, your child may need an extra sandwich or other snack in the winter months because hunger is higher due to the body burning more calories to keep warm.

Introduce more meat and hot dishes such as soups, cooked vegetables and grains on a daily basis. Salad is a great side dish. Hot stewed fruits, such as apples and pears, are simple to prepare and easy to digest. Mild spices such as turmeric, chilli, garlic and cooked onions can be introduced to your child in this season in roast dinners, Asian-style dishes and casseroles.

Keep up the dose of vitamin C – half a teaspoon of children's vitamin C powder twice a day – especially if your child is prone to coughs and colds (see chapter 1). If your child is constantly coming down with bronchial problems, make sure you visit a naturopath or herbalist for advice.

Your herbalist or naturopath can make the following herbal tonic for you to help boost your child's immunity and prevent colds and bronchial problems: echinacea (40 per cent), thyme (10 per cent), astragalus (20 per cent), marshmallow (20 per cent), peppermint (5 per cent) and liquorice (5 per cent). Give 1 teaspoon once a day in half a glass of warm water with half a teaspoon of honey.

# Spring

Spring is said to be the most beautiful season in the calendar year because it heralds new birth for animals and flowers and new growth to fruits, berries and vegetables. Fittingly, it is a time to change your child's diet to include lighter foods, to detox the body from the heavier winter carbohydrates and proteins, and prepare the mind and body for new concentration, thinking and development. But spring also brings fresh pollens into the air, which can aggravate a histamine reaction and cause runny noses and sneezing allergies.

If your child suffers from allergies, give them fresh orange and pineapple juice daily, for the vitamin C and bioflavonoid content. Also, introduce a tea made from a herb called eyebright (euphrasia) mixed with peppermint; for children aged over eight, give 2–3 cups daily. In the evenings, put a few drops of peppermint oil or eucalyptus oil on your child's pillow before they go to bed. The menthol property in peppermint helps inhibit nasal symptoms such as sneezing and blocked noses.

If your child suffers from itchy eyes, use moisturising drops from your pharmacy; 1–2 drops in the eyes twice daily.

Begin to introduce new tastes to your child's diet, with different types of vegetables, particularly green leafy vegetables with olive oil and honey dressing. (You can toss walnuts and crushed almonds through these salads.)

Try cranberry juice as a new taste for spring; this juice helps prevent bacterial infections in children. Diluted carrot juice is also good for its natural vitamin A content, which strengthens the mucosa in the lining of the nasal passageways.

Some of my herbal teas are designed to cleanse the digestive system and are delicious to taste. Try Lemon Tang (a mixture of lemongrass and peppermint), Berry Tea (it tastes like fresh berry juice without the sugar) and Summer Delight (a mixture of mints that assist sinus and the springtime runny nose – also see pages 126–30).

# 9
# Nutrition and weight control

In the twenty-first century we are facing a dramatically increasing problem of overweight children, which is often referred to as 'childhood obesity'.

If you need to confirm whether your child's weight is normal or dangerous, consult your doctor. They can talk to you about your child's Body Mass Index (BMI), which is an international measurement, adjusted for age and sex, to calculate obesity. A child is classed as obese if their BMI exceeds the cut-off point for their age. Your doctor can also show you standard growth charts and measures of fat for children.

When considering a child's nutrition and weight, a naturopath will check the child's nutritional intake against their physical activity and leisure time. A thorough case history plus a food diary will be taken to assess the lifestyle patterns of the child.

Unfortunately, an increase in children's sedentary activities such as computers, video games, television and transportation by car, train or bus without enough physical activity can all lead to excess weight. Also, children are eating many more sugary snacks, fizzy drinks and often high-fat takeaway food due to peer pressure or the fact that both parents work long hours.

Often the treatment or preventative program for an overweight child can be simple and rewarding, and children can play an active part with the preparation of food. Here is an example of a program you can try.

## Treatment

- Throw out all chocolate, sweets and sugary snacks and replace with fresh fruits, honey, brown sugars and low-fat ice-creams.

- Start introducing complex carbohydrates, which take longer to break down into sugars and therefore do not cause insulin surges. These include brown rice, couscous, buckwheat and wholemeal grainy breads.

- Prepare healthy snacks for your child to eat when they come home from school (your child can help with the preparation). This could be a toasted sandwich filled with a tin of tuna or chunks of avocado, a homemade vegetable soup, a bowl of cereal or hot porridge, an omelette or a boiled egg on toast. Then serve a fresh fruit to follow, and a handful of nuts and raisins.

- Set time for watching television or computer work, and encourage your child to participate in a local sport they love, or even gym work.

- Instead of driving, walk with your child to school or to the bus stop.

- Make sure your child drinks water, freshly squeezed juices and herbal teas daily for fluid intake and circulation.

> ### Sugar cravings
>
> A tonic made from equal parts of fenugreek, dandelion root, liquorice, gymnea and peppermint is an excellent way to assist overweight children control their sugar cravings. These herbs are a tonic for the liver and pancreas; gymnea (an Indian herb) is used successfully for insulin imbalances and diabetes in adults and (in smaller doses) for children. Give 2.5 ml in water three times a day for three to four months.

# ❈ Basic foods

## Grains

The following grains can be incorporated into your child's diet over time.

Barley can be used two to three times a week in soups or as a base for stews. This grain is highly nutritious and gives long-lasting energy. Barley can be used in cooked cereals with cracked wheat or as flour to make pancakes. Barley water mixed with fruit juice is wonderful for building up your child's strength, particularly children who are very active or have a strenuous physical routine. It is also excellent for girls who suffer urinary tract infections.

Buckwheat is an underrated grain that provides strength and energy. Buckwheat is native to central Asia and is not really classed as a wheat grain. Try using it instead of rice; to make a meal add the vegetables and protein of your choice and finish with soy sauce. Buckwheat flour tastes nutty, and children love it for pancakes and rolled sandwiches.

Many children, especially those with high allergy levels, are allergic to cornflour. If your child is not allergic, cornflour can be used for thickening sauces and making light breads.

Millet is not particularly nice-tasting, and children often do not like it unless it is mixed as flour to use for breads or pancakes. Millet is gluten-free, so children with celiac disease need to regularly eat this grain with rice.

Oats are an underused grain. Oats contain wonderful active ingredients to sooth the nervous system and build stamina. Use oats in porridge and cookies, and use oat flakes in cereals or any grain dish.

Wheat is the most widely grown grain in the world. There are five classes of wheat: hard red spring, soft red winter, hard red winter, durum and white. Durum wheat is used in macaroni, spaghetti and noodles. This grain is lighter that the cracked grain of the harder kernels, and children often prefer the lighter durum wheat. Children who are allergic to wheat can often eat rye breads. Rye is a heavier grain than wheat, and it is great for a snack with a protein on top. Rye is much more popular in eastern Mediterranean countries where it grows.

Rice, originating in South-East Asia, has been cultivated for over 4000 years. There are many varieties of rice, depending on the size of the grain, such as long or short. The outer bran is removed in the processing of white rice, whereas it is kept in brown rice; brown rice therefore has better fibre and nutrient content. Sometimes children find brown rice difficult to digest, so cook it thoroughly and mix it with white rice.

# Honey

The darker, pure varieties of honey offer the best nutritional value, and children should have them instead of white sugars on pancakes, in milk drinks and on fruits.

The sugars in honey can be easily absorbed in the blood stream. Honey often satisfies sugar cravings in children and has a cleansing antiseptic effect on the blood stream. Children can gargle honey to soothe a sore throat, and honey can also be spread over scratches and any small ulcer-like cuts.

Remember, honey has been highly acclaimed throughout history for its powerful healing abilities, so why not use it each day for your child instead of sugar-filled lollies? Buying bee pollen with fresh honey is a nice way to give your child a sweet treat.

# Berries

Dark berries such as blackberries, blueberries, cranberries, blackcurrants, elderberries, mulberries, loganberries and strawberries all contain high levels of vitamin C and antioxidants necessary for children's health.

Berries help regulate children's bowel motions. Cranberry juice is also a wonderful treatment for cystitis, keeping bacterial infections under control.

Research is being undertaken in Germany regarding the role of blueberries, blackberries and raspberries in controlling non-insulin diabetes. This is especially relevant for children who may have a susceptibility to sugar dependence and being overweight.

The great news is that children generally love berries because they are sweet. You can use them as a desert with yoghurt and honey, or put them in homemade muffins or biscuits for a delicious and nutritious snack. Fresh berry juices from health food stores can be used with water for children's drinks instead of fizzy sugar drinks that contain added colourings.

> **Macrobiotic cooking**
>
> I strongly recommend all parents invest in a good macrobiotic health cookbook – this will help you understand the best ways to cook and serve grains and legumes for your child. Ask your health food store for a recommendation.

# Legumes

Introduce your child slowly to the basic legumes – such as lima beans, adzuki beans and black-eyed beans – in soups, spreads and casseroles.

Chickpeas can be enjoyed in casseroles with vegetables served on rice, or crushed (and mixed with a little olive oil) to make a hummus spread for sandwiches or a dip served with raw vegetables.

Baby kidney beans (adzuki beans) can be served in soups and casseroles, and can be mixed with mashed pumpkin or potato for a nutritious dinner vegetable. They can also be introduced to children with couscous and vegetables.

Lima beans, when cooked and mashed with a little butter, oil and salt, taste like mashed potatoes. You can mix them with mashed potato or mashed sweet pumpkin and serve with chicken, red meat or salad.

Children do not seem to take a liking to most other beans. However, if you have an adventurous child, introduce them to soy and black-eyed beans; try them in minestrone soup.

## ✺ Herbal teas

Herbal teas can play a vital role in the prevention and treatment of ailments in children.

As a herbalist and naturopath, I have created a range of organic loose-leaf teas that help my clients increase their daily fluid intake as well as prevent and soothe common ailments affecting the digestive and nervous systems. These teas also help carry nutrients around the body and stimulate the excretion of wastes from the blood.

These teas are safe for children; in fact, children can have 3–4 cups a day. When used with the recommendations in this book, herbal teas are very therapeutic for children. Herbal teas can be used in a number of ways: as a warm tea drink, an iced tea in summer, or even in iceblock form. Herbal teas are also a great substitute for fizzy drinks filled with sugar, preservatives and colourings; and, all herbal teas can be sweetened with honey to taste.

Only buy herbal tea in the organic loose-leaf form, for its healing effects. The tea in herbal tea bags is generally ground down to a powder and has therefore lost the essential oil that is needed in the healing effect of the tea. They may have a nice taste through added flavourings, but they will not have the therapeutic value required.

All of my herbal teas are organic loose-leaf and grown in Australia. Use the following guide to assist your choice.

- **Apres** contains chamomile, fennel, aniseed and peppermint. This tea is highly suitable for those who suffer anxiety, stress, poor digestion, heartburn and mild insomnia. Chamomile has traditionally been used to soothe colic, upset stomachs in adults and frayed nerves. Fennel, aniseed and peppermint all aid poor digestion and help calm an aggravated stomach.

- **Berry** contains hawthorn berries, elderberries and juniper berries. Hawthorn berry assists circulatory problems and has antioxidant properties. Elderberries and juniper berries assist the sweet taste of this natural herbal tea.

- **Lemon Tang** contains lemongrass and peppermint. This tea is ideal after fatty meals to help in the digestive process. It is cooling and soothing in hot weather and assists with kidney function.

- **Petal** contains organic red clover, lemongrass, lavender, rose petals and chamomile. This tea assists in cleaning the blood. Red clover has been used throughout history as a blood purifier. Lemongrass assists in stimulating the kidneys and therefore works as a mild diuretic, decreasing fluid retention. Lavender, chamomile and rose petals are known to be calmative plants, relaxing and healing for those who suffer stress and anxiety.

- **Summer Delight** contains organic spearmint, peppermint, lemongrass and aniseed. This minty tea is ideal for assisting digestion by stimulating digestive enzymes and relaxing and calming the body. Peppermint has a long history of aiding digestion of fish and meat dishes. This tea is ideal after any meal.

- **Triple E** contains liquorice root, aniseed, fennel and peppermint. This tea has a profound healing effect on the bowel and stomach, helping with sluggishness and heartburn. Pure liquorice root works as a mild anti-inflammatory, hence liquorice is used in most cough medicine and laxative-type medication.

# Dos and don'ts

**Do**: Introduce your child to herbal teas with a little honey or brown sugar if they like something sweet; or introduce teas by adding half a cup to a milk drink.

**Do**: Make the tea weaker at first by only using 1 teaspoon to 2 cups of boiling water.

**Do**: Initially serve herbal teas to your child lukewarm.

**Do**: Use reliable organic brands – check with your local health food store.

**Do**: Make herbal iceblocks with honey. Mimic commercial iceblocks by making them with two sticks; or form in animal shapes (you can buy these shapes in trays).

**Don't**: Use fresh herbs from the garden unless you know them well and they are recommended in this book or by a herbalist.

**Don't**: Insist that your child drink the herbal tea undiluted. Try different ways of introducing teas as recommended above.

# 10
# A child's healthy diet

To help keep your child healthy, happy and ailment-free, I have set out a basic healthy diet for children aged between five and twelve.

Naturally, there will be foods in this diet your child does not like. The most important thing to remember is to work with the foods your child does like, even if you have to serve them on a daily basis. It is better for your child to eat the same, good-quality foods all the time than to eat junk foods or, worse still, to not eat at all.

### CASE STUDY

An eight-year-old boy, Mario, came into my clinic with his parents because he was not eating anything they prepared for him; he was so thin, it was frightening to see. Mario only liked to eat McDonald's and had not eaten anything at all for the past five days. The parents said no to McDonald's but they failed to realise that they had started a battle of psychological stamina on both sides.

I asked Mario what food he loved best; he told me he loved spaghetti bolognaise but was not allowed to eat it. I explained to the parents that the meat in this dish had proteins to build the body, and the tomato contained high levels of vitamin C and lycopene (an active ingredient that has antioxidant properties).

I asked Mario's parents to give him spaghetti bolognaise for breakfast, lunch and dinner each day, and to take him to McDonald's once a week for the next three weeks. I also prescribed 1 multivitamin tablet once a day with a herbal iron tonic (1 teaspoon twice a day), because he was anaemic.

I knew that after three weeks Mario would be eating all sorts of foods the family presented. Exactly two weeks later I received a phone call from the parents saying that Mario was so fed up with spaghetti bolognaise that he was eating fish, chicken and some vegetables. He felt sick in the stomach at McDonald's (because he now had some good foods in his system) and he was gaining weight.

I have often seen parents insisting on foods their child does not want to eat or foods the child protests against; then, weakening, sweets and lollies are given to the child to keep them quiet. The best option for parents is to choose the vegetables and proteins their child likes and make sure they eat these ones regularly before giving any dessert or sweet. A healthy milkshake with fresh fruit, yoghurt and protein powder is a wonderful snack.

Often children will love simple things such as mashed potatoes, and in this you can hide other mashed vegetables. Children often also like frozen peas; if this is the only vegetable they like, give it to them every night until their taste buds are mature enough for more variety.

Many children dislike fish, because it is often too oily for their undeveloped digestive systems. If this is the case with your child, choose fish that does not have bones and is not too oily (your fishmonger can help you with your selection). To make fish more appetising for your child, crumb it and sauté in a small amount of oil and butter; this, served with their favourite vegetable and/or salad, is a perfect meal. You can also hide the 'fishy' taste by making fish patties mixed with rice or couscous.

Make sure there is no junk food in your pantry for your child to help themselves to when hungry. Try to follow the snack ideas in this book (see pages 142–5) so your child always has a homemade, healthy snack or meal available. Children often go straight from school to a sporting activity, and they need extra nourishment; I recommend parents bring snacks from home such as a sandwich, rice salad or even a milkshake if they are collecting their children. This is the easiest time of the day for children to fill up on sugary foods, resulting in irritability and low energy for study. So it is worth your while to prepare healthy, sugar-free after-school snacks – you will have more peace and better performance from your child.

Children often throw out their lunch if they do not like the food, and they will very rarely tell their parents. Ask your child to give you an idea of their favourite three lunches, and rotate them each day. For example, if your child requests a vegemite sandwich, this has no long-lasting food value; tell your child they can have this sandwich for recess but must choose a protein (that won't make the bread soggy) on their sandwich for lunch. Proteins such as chicken, ham, red meat, legumes or cheese (choose a good-quality white cheese) are ideal. Again, work on what your child does like and grow slowly from there.

You don't have to change everything at once, but if you introduce the principles in this book, you will find a happier and a healthier child.

# A child's healthy diet

## Breakfast

- Freshly squeezed orange juice or sliced fruit.

- A high-quality yoghurt with acidophilus (the good bacteria).

- Muesli or porridge, or a cereal that does not have a lot of added sugar and preservatives. A favourite fruit can be put on the top.

- Choose from the following list of protein breakfasts and rotate them each morning:
  - wholemeal toast with poached or scrambled eggs, baked beans or tinned tuna or sardines
  - wholemeal toast with avocado and white cheese (ricotta, fetta or goat's cheese)

- wholemeal toast with a spread such as vegemite, nut paste or hummus.

- An omelette filled with the previous night's vegetables, or fresh tomato and capsicum.

- Pancakes (wholemeal, buckwheat or rice flour) with fruit and honey, or a savoury pancake with eggs or vegetables such as tomato, capsicum or avocado.

## Morning tea (or recess at school)

- Wholemeal biscuits with a spread of nuts, vegemite or cheese.

- A handful of almonds, cashews or macadamias with a small amount of dried fruits.

- A fresh fruit such as a banana, apple or pear.

- A mini-sandwich (one piece of bread filled and rolled over).

- A cold pancake filled with a vegetable, hummus or light meat.

## Lunch

- One to three sandwiches (children will often require more sandwiches when they are going through a growing spurt, which is often around the age of eight or nine) filled with a protein, such as chicken, red meat, ham, fish (this can be wrapped separately so it doesn't make the bread soggy), cheese and legume paste (hummus or nut paste).

- Cut-up raw vegetables such as carrots, celery, capsicum and cucumber.

- Rice or couscous salad with a protein and vegetable.

- A thermos of hot, thick chicken and vegetable soup, or minestrone soup with legumes.

- A pasta dish with a bolognaise sauce (from the previous

night's dinner) or a pasta with the child's favourite topping (this must include a protein).

## Afternoon tea

- Toasted sandwich.

- Thick soup (made with vegetables and a protein such as chicken, meat or legumes).

- Wholemeal bread with avocado or tinned fish such as tuna, salmon or sardines.

- Milkshake with fruits and protein powder (available from health food stores).

- Wholemeal biscuits with a spread such as nut paste, fish paste, tuna, salmon, chicken, ham or egg on top.

- Fruit (fresh or stewed) and yoghurt.

- A slice of wholemeal bread or a cracker topped with honey.

## Dinner

- Fish, chicken or meat accompanied by three vegetables of different colours, such as green (lettuce, peas, broccoli, zucchini, rocket, string beans), orange (pumpkin, carrots, sweet potato) and white (potatoes, cauliflower, cucumber, cabbage).

- Children love stirfries and casseroles, so try different ways of cooking meat and vegetables (even add tofu and legumes if your child likes them) and serve them on a grain base or a carbohydrate such as pasta, rice or buckwheat.

- A roast dinner – always a favourite with children and very easy to prepare.

- Chicken or red meat baked with root vegetables such as potato, pumpkin, parsnip, sweet potato, onion and garlic.

Serve with a steamed green vegetable such as broccoli, peas or spinach, or a green salad.

- Rice and egg noodles with proteins and lots of vegetables.

## Dessert

- Soy ice-cream with fresh or stewed fruit.

- Yoghurt with fresh or stewed fruit.

- Homemade apple crumble with yoghurt or soy ice-cream.

- Homemade dark chocolate cookie (dark chocolate is better that light chocolate because dark chocolate contains no dairy and is higher in a substance called theobromine, which is found in all chocolate and works as a bronchial dilator).

- Whole apples or pears baked with a cinnamon stick and a little honey for flavour.

## Supper

▦ Yoghurt or a glass of warm milk with a little honey; you can add half a cup of chamomile tea to the mix to assist sleep.

> ### Lunch-box ideas
>
> When preparing a healthy, well-balanced and delicious lunch box for your child to take to school, follow these steps.
> 1. Include an item from the lunch menu.
> 2. Include an item from the morning and afternoon tea menus.
> 3. Include two pieces of fruit.
> 4. Include either slices of your child's favourite raw vegetable with a small container of hummus to dip, or celery sticks filled with cream cheese.
> 5. Include yoghurt and pure fruit juice.
> 6. For something different, add a special treat from the following list.
>    - a sushi roll or sushi ball

- a protein or muesli bar
- a slice of natural honeycomb
- a honey or chocolate crackle
- a carob bar
- some sugar- and preservative-free jubes
- a liquorice sweet
- a square of dark chocolate.

# Healthy, nutritious snacks – getting back to basics

It is so much better to spend half a day each week preparing snacks to freeze for your child than to give them pocket money to buy snacks outside the home. In the cupboard at home make sure you have a sandwich toaster and a milkshake maker or blender. Remember: it is better that your child has a mini-dinner in the afternoon and a smaller dinner in the evening than to fill up on junk foods or sweets. Even if they are playing sport after school, they can take extra food or prepare the following simple food at home.

- Toasted sandwiches filled with tuna, salmon, tomato or cheese (or other preferred vegetables).

- If your child is allergic to dairy, make milkshakes with soy, goat's or rice milk. Fruits, yoghurt and ground nuts are always great in a milkshake. You can also use a good protein powder, which adds extra nutrition if your child is a poor eater yet loves milkshakes. For a special treat, add a scoop of soy ice-cream.

- Soups served with wholemeal toast are a great snack, especially in winter. You can freeze the soup and take it from the freezer in the morning.

- If you are around to supervise cooking, help your child prepare a homemade hamburger of red meat or chicken with slices of fresh tomato and some lettuce.

- A bowl of fresh fruit and yoghurt.

- Cereal with fruit (fresh or stewed) and yoghurt, or a bowl of hot porridge in winter.

- An omelette filled with cheese and tomato, capsicum or mushrooms – whatever healthy fillings your child loves.

- Pancakes with a fruit or savoury topping.

> **A note on fruit and bar snacks**
>
> Muesli bars, protein bars and other sorts of bars have become popular with children. Unfortunately, these bars have replaced good-quality homemade soups, sandwiches and rice dishes.
>
> Bars are often filled with colourings and preservatives, and in fact many children are not only allergic to nuts (especially asthmatic and eczematous children; in many Australian schools, children are no longer allowed to bring nuts in any

form to school), but the bars can be very difficult to digest. The added colourings can cause a child to be more hyperactive.

Only use these bars sparingly and make sure you do some research on the labels. These bars will never replace homemade snacks for good nutrition.

# 11
# Common childhood issues

## ✸ Thumb-sucking

Often this happens at an early age, particularly if a child has a special blanket to take to bed or is just using their thumb for a comfort to go to sleep.

Thumb-sucking can become a problem if it continues after your child starts school – they may be teased by their peers and feel inadequate, which can result in mood swings and anxiety.

You can buy nasty-tasting pastes that can be applied to the thumb regularly to stop the habit. It is also important to introduce reward systems as your child breaks the habit. Often a dentist can suggest ideas and also have a look at the structure of your child's mouth to make sure there is no long-term damage to the palate.

# Head lice

Lice are widespread in schools; you must therefore be regular and diligent in observing your child – any signs of an itchy scalp must be examined. Using shampoo and conditioner on your child's hair, and then combing through it while wet, is a must (use a comb, not a brush). Tea tree oil shampoos used regularly stop many recurrences of lice, and a few drops of rosemary and lavender oil rubbed into the scalp regularly stops the infestation and assists the control of lice. Direct application of these essential oils can burn your child's scalp, so put the few drops of each into your child's conditioner.

# Thrush and an inflamed vagina in girls

This problem can occur particularly between the ages of five and twelve. Symptoms include a red, itchy vagina and, sometimes, a white discharge. This problem can occur when girls touch their vaginal area (often because of stress or anxiety) or regularly wet the bed – an infection and aggravation from the acidic urine can cause a red inflamed area, sometimes without the discharge.

Encourage your child not to touch her vaginal area. Also teach her to wipe herself properly after using her bowel and bladder, and to wash the area with a gentle soap and water each day. If your child is suffering from thrush, it is a good idea to clean the vaginal and anal area with anti-bacterial cloth wipes each time your child goes to the toilet, in order to stop the faecal bacteria moving into these areas. Acidophilus powder with a few drops of water used as a paste around the vagina twice daily is wonderfully soothing to the inflamed area. Paw paw cream used through the day is also gentle and can help relieve symptoms.

# Foreskin health for boys

Small infections can occur under the foreskin of boys who are not circumcised. It is imperative for parents, particularly a father, to show a child how to pull back the foreskin of the penis and wash this area each morning under the shower, in order to prevent infection. If your child is self-conscious about this area, take him to a trusted doctor (preferably male) and ask him to show your child how to go about the care of this delicate area.

## ❈ Urinary tract infections

This is rare in children, but occasionally children pick up this infection or some bacterial infection in pools.

A good-quality cranberry juice (from your health food store) is excellent in healing this infection. You can also boil up barley water for your child, and give them 1 teaspoon of echinacea a day, and 1 garlic oil tablet each morning and evening until the infection abates. Encourage your child to drink water regularly.

## ❈ Teeth care

Insist that your child clean their teeth each morning and evening, and ask your dentist to show your child the correct methods for maintaining healthy gums – correct motions of the toothbrush are important, and many children worsen their gums through heavy circular motions. If your child complains of sore gums, ask your dentist for a treatment, and cut back on all acidic fruits such as pineapple, oranges and lemons, as well as vinegars, refined sugars and vitamin C powders. If your child is supplementing with vitamin C, make sure they clean their teeth after taking the powder. If your child is not having dairy products, supplement with 1 child's calcium, magnesium and mineral tablet per day.

## Worms

This problem often occurs in children who regularly spend time around animals or on farms, or do not wash their hands after each toilet visit. Threadworms are the most common variety, and symptoms include an itchy anus and the child boring their fingers into their nostrils.

Your doctor can recommend a short treatment course for the entire family to take (worms are easily passed on to other members of the family). I recommend 1 garlic oil capsule twice a day and a herb called black walnut (see your herbalist for the appropriate dose).

## Nail-biting

This is a frequent problem with children who are anxious or nervy, especially if their home environment is a little unsettled or they have problems at school.

In all my experience with this problem I have found that treating the child for nerves is a great help (see chapter 5), as well as regular manicures, which cut away dead skin tissue and keep the cuticles strong. You can buy pastes for your child's fingers – these pastes taste awful in order to help your child break the habit. You can also use a nail hardener. Make sure your child's intake of calcium is adequate – if it is not, supplement with a child's mineral powder or tablet for internal nail strength.

## Hygiene

Often this issue is obvious, but unfortunately it is sometimes not followed through with children aged between five and twelve. Parents think their child is washing their hands regularly after the toilet or wiping themselves correctly, but children can be lazy and are often rushing to other activities and forget to wash their hands.

To help your child maintain strong personal hygiene, insist they wash their hands with soap and water after every visit to the bathroom, and give some rewards for the effort your child puts into this important life habit.

# ✱ Sore and dry eyes

Children often have dry and sore eyes around seasonal changes. If this is the case with your child, I recommend you buy some moisture drops from your local chemist to place in your child's eyes each morning and evening. These drops are especially useful for children (and adults) who are going to drier climates and to the mountains for snow skiing.

# How to buy supplements

When choosing supplements, there are some very simple guidelines to follow. It is important to be aware of these guidelines to ensure that you experience what good-quality medicinal herbs and therapeutic vitamins can do for your child's vitality and health.

There are many brands of vitamins and herbs in health food stores and pharmacies – all of different qualities and prices – and it is very difficult to know exactly what you should buy. In this book I have given general dosages for each condition so you know what to look for. However, I always recommend that you visit a qualified, registered naturopath, herbalist, nutritionist or health consultant in order to get the most out of supplements and complementary therapies.

Tell them as much as you can about your child's medical history and lifestyle. Make notes before your visit. Your child may recently have had a blood test that is relevant – make sure you take along the results if known. Also take along any medication they are taking, as well as any vitamins or complementary medicines. It is vital that your practitioner knows about any medications your child is on from your doctor so they can discuss any contraindications in relation to your vitamins and herbs. They can sort out if they are suitable in dosage and quality and also check on expiry dates.

Your practitioner is trained to know the correct therapeutic doses for your child, depending on their condition, body weight, age and height. Your practitioner also knows which products have quality standards and in-depth sourcing standards. If you are buying supplements and are unsure about the information on the label, you should ring the information line (the number should be on the label) to ask about the company's sourcing and quality standards. If this information is refused, do not buy the product, and again see your naturopath or trusted health food store to guide you to suitable brands.

The key words to look out for on labels of herbal medicine are 'standardised extract'. The standardised extract tells you how much of the active ingredient (the medicinal part) is present in that particular supplement. For example, a label for echinacea supplements should say that you are taking 600 mg of echinacea root, containing alkyamides 2.65 mg (the active ingredient). Research was carried out on several echinacea products in the market to see if they contained the active ingredient of alkyamides (from the echinacea root). Three of these products did not use the echinacea root at all and three other products did not contain any active ingredient. So be sure to check the label.

If you are giving your child any form of complementary medicine for the first time, start by giving one medication at a time and see if there is improvement over a period of three weeks. You may then wish to introduce another recommended supplement for the next three weeks. If your child does not improve, there can be a few obvious reasons:

- Your child is not taking (or you are not administering) the prescribed dose in accordance with your practitioner's instructions or the advice on the label.

- If you are following correct dosages for your child, the medicine is either not suitable or you need to give the medication another month to see the effect. In this case you can check with your health consultant.

- If you have prescribed medicines for your child, the quality or quantity of the medicine may be incorrect for your child's body size and weight. Check this with your health consultant.

If your child does not feel well with any supplement, stop giving it immediately and check with your consultant. Remember that any concentrated medicine, whether pharmaceutical or complementary, generally needs to be taken with food. Also, do not allow your child to take medicines before bed unless prescribed that way. Vary your child's medicines. Have some as tablets, and some as powders and liquids.

# Conclusion

Our world is changing rapidly, as are our children's thoughts, beliefs and ability to take an active role in their health and wellbeing. There are now many influences outside the home that affect the physical and mental wellbeing of our future generations. Life has never moved so quickly, and with this increased tempo we are seeing many more 'fast' influences, such as fast-food chains, fast-moving computers and fast-moving technology to which even our small children at school are introduced.

It has never been more important to teach our 'little people' good values in life, and show them the importance of quiet meditative time, exercise and fresh air, and respect for what they eat. Our children need to understand the challenges they will face in building their small body to a healthy, happy and balanced individual – if we can teach them the importance of respect for their bodies and minds, we will nourish them and the environment in which they live. We will have done a great service towards maintaining the peace, happiness and understanding of our planet.

Throughout my sixteen years of clinical work I have been continually rewarded by seeing these wonderful attributes develop in children. I have seen many children whom I began treating at the age of five or six and who are now teenagers, stand with confidence and realise that they are indeed what they eat, and that anything is possible in life if you encompass good health, regular exercise and a positive mental outlook. In fact, many of the teenagers I treat remember the 'nasty-tasting tonics' they took as children that made them feel so much better; they remember the herbs and vitamins that helped them through difficult times with their asthma; they remember the minerals they took to help them through various growth spurts – but most of all they tell me they simply enjoy feeling healthy. They ask their parents to bring them to see me for a 'little problem' and insist they would rather deal with it 'the natural way'.

These children already understand that through natural healing they are building their bodies, cells, minds and positive attitudes. These children always surprise me with their commonsense and eagerness to 'feel fantastic'. They enjoy learning about food and herbs; they enjoy learning about their health; and they especially enjoy learning what it is that gives star sportspeople their strength and how Mum and Dad stay fit. This is where the importance of role-modelling comes in.

Our children are our future, and it is through them that our understanding of natural medicine will reach further and merge with our approach to life and wellbeing. I believe that in the not-too-distant future, natural medicine will become a way of life for health and vitality, with Western medicine taking its appropriate place for illnesses that do not rapidly respond to ongoing preventative health care.

There is still so much to be done to educate our children, our society and ourselves in healthier ways of living, but I certainly hope this book will give you some inspiration for our truly beautiful children. Remember, along with good food and natural medicine, the most important things for children are fresh air and fun. Enjoy your children – each and every one of them has special potential and deserves the best you can give them. Enjoy every moment of your child's development; children are our future, our strength, our inspiration and our greatest happiness.

# Index

abdominal pain 97
acidic foods 89
acidophilus
    and antibiotics 33, 47
    for bowel problems 101, 107
    for vaginal infection 148
active ingredient in supplements 154–5
additives in food 12, 25, 50, 56, 96, 97
adenoids 41, 44
ADHD 54–67
adzuki beans 125
allergies
    and asthma 24–7
    in autumn and spring 111, 115
    and immune system 10
    *see also* food allergies
aloe vera juice 101
anaemia 21, 95
*Andrographis paniculate* 20
animal hair 26
antibiotics 10, 32, 43–4, 46–7
antibodies 20
antioxidants 12, 13, 51, 63
antiseptic effect of honey 123
anxiety 52, 68–74, 128
appetite 79
apples 104, 110
Apres herbal tea 127
artificial additives *see* colourings in food; additives in food
aspirin allergy 56
asthma 24–35

Attention Deficit Hyperactivity Disorder 54–67
autumn 27, 111–12

bacopa 52, 53, 64
bacterial infection 20, 37, 124
bananas 29, 109
barley 120–1, 149
bars as snacks 144–5
baths 81, 92
bedwetting 53, 148
berries 123–4
Berry herbal tea 128
bioflavonoids 12
black tea 104
blocked nose 15, 16, 18, 115
Body Mass Index 117
bowel flora 32–3
bowel movements 98–9, 124
brain 12, 48–67
bread 16, 59, 99, 100
breakfast ideas
    ADHD diet 60–1
    to aid concentration 50–1
    when child has eczema 89
    for general health 135–6
    for improved digestion 100
    in winter 113
bronchial problems 15, 26
brown rice 100, 122
buckwheat 121

calcium 71, 84
carrot juice 115–16
chamomile 77
    creams 91
    essential oil 72

    tea 40, 65–6, 77, 98
    tincture 53
chemicals and ADHD 58
chickpeas 125
chickweed ointment 90, 93
chocolate 140
cinnamon 105
cod liver oil 23, 31, 51
colds 15–21
colic 65, 77, 127
colourings in food 50, 56, 71, 97–8
complex carbohydrates 118
computer use 76, 118
concentration problems 49–54
constipation 98–102
cordial 12
cornflour 121
cortisone cream 86, 93
coughs 15, 21
cranberry juice 115, 124, 149
cystitis 124

dairy products
    allergy testing 89
    alternatives 28, 84
    and asthma 25
    for calcium 84
    and immune system 16, 41
dehydration 17, 103, 109
depression 67, 72
dessert ideas 74, 140
detox diets 65, 114–15
diabetes 120, 124
diarrhoea 19, 47, 102–6
diet 75–6
    for ADHD 60–3

for general health 131–45
*see also* food diary
digestive system 66, 95–107, 128
dinner ideas 62–3, 139–40
dopamine 56–7
dosages 8, 155–6
dried fruits 29
dry eyes 152
durum wheat 122
dust mites 24–5, 90

earaches 36–42
echinacea 13, 16, 18–19, 155
eczema 77, 86–94
eggs 89
electrolytes 109
emotional problems 26, 53
eucalyptus 18, 40
evening primrose oil 91
eyebright 115
eyes, sore 152
exercise
    and asthma 33–5
    and weight control 119

fibre 98, 99, 100, 106
fish 11, 110, 112, 133
fizzy drinks
    and ADHD 58
    and immune system 12
    and restlessness 76
    substitutes for 107, 127
flavonoids 104
flu 15–23
fluid intake 17, 126
folic acid 48–9
food allergies
    in ADHD 56
    in asthma 24, 25–6
    cornflour 121
    in digestive problems 97–8
food diary
    for restlessness 75–6
    for skin conditions 87, 88
    for stomach upsets 98
foreskin 148–9

fruit juices 12, 108–9, 115
fruits 12, 51

gargle 105
garlic 39, 65, 149, 150
ginkgo 53
glands 9, 10
glue ear 37–8
glycetracts 14
goat's milk yoghurt 30
grains 120–2
green vegetables 13
grommets 37, 38
growing pains 83–5
growth spurts 76
gum problems 105, 150
gymnea 120

hair lice 147
hawthorn berry 128
headaches 72
hearing problems 36, 37
heavy foods 16, 111–12
heavy metals 55, 65
herbal teas 116, 126–30 *see also* specific herbal teas
herbalists 153–4
herbs for healing 3–4, 7 *see also* specific herb names
holistic treatment 68
homoscyteine 49
honey 44–5, 103, 123
hydration *see* dehydration
hygiene 148, 151–2
hyperactivity 49, 51, 56, 66 *see also* ADHD
hyperventilation 25

iceblocks 130
immune system 9–23, 38, 102, 108
infections 19, 20
    ear and tonsil 36, 37, 38
    sinus 15, 36
insomnia 52, 72
iron 21, 105
irritability 72
itchy anus 150

itchy eyes 115
itchy scalp 147
itchy skin 90–2

juice 12, 101, 108–9, 115

kidney function 128

lavender oil 72, 91
learning difficulties 43
legumes 29–30, 59, 90, 125–6
lemon juice 17
Lemon Tang herbal tea 128
lemongrass 128
lice 147
light foods 16, 110
lima beans 126
liquorice root 129
liver 12, 63, 64–5
lunch box ideas 141–2
lunch ideas 61–2, 137–8
lymph glands 9

macrobiotic cooking 125
magnesium 78, 105
mashed potato 133
medicines, taking 155–6 *see also* antibiotics
memory 53
milk 71 *see also* dairy products
milkshakes 133
millet 121
minerals 66, 72, 80
mouth ulcers 105
mucous 31, 32, 39 *see also* phlegm
muesli bars 144–5
multivitamins 22, 49, 52

nail-biting 151
naturopaths 117, 153–4
nausea 73
nerve cells 51
nutrition 117–30
nutritionists 117, 153–4
nuts 29, 144–5

oats 92, 103, 121–2

# index

obesity 117
omega 3 and 6 oils 11, 31, 51, 53, 64, 92
onions 21, 39
orange fruits 12
orange vegetables 13
osteopaths 84

pancakes 110
passionflower 53, 72
paw paw cream 148
peanuts 29
peppermint
  oil 115
  tea 16, 70, 129
Petal herbal tea 128
phlegm 15, 16 *see also* mucous
pinetarsol 91
pollen 26, 111, 115
porridge 103
pregnancy 48-9
preservatives in food 12, 25, 56, 96
protein 11, 29-30, 84
protein bars 145
prunes 101
psyllium husks 100, 101
pumpkin seeds 13

rashes 25, 86-94
raspberry leaf tea 105
Rast test, for allergies 25, 93
recess snacks 136-7
refined foods 12
Rescue Remedy 78
restlessness 74-83
rice 100, 103, 122
rice water 106
Ritalin 56-7
runny nose 15-16, 115
rye 122

salicylates 56
salt 109
salt water spray 18
sandwich ideas 61, 134, 137

schisandra 63, 64
sinus problems 15, 36
skin conditions 86-94
sleep 53-4, 69 *see also* insomnia; sleeplessness
sleeplessness 79 *see also* insomnia
slippery elm 104
smoking 48, 55
snack ideas
  for ADHD children 61
  after school 119, 142-4
  afternoon tea 138-9
  for asthmatic children 28
  milkshakes 133, 143
  morning tea 136-7
  in winter 113
sodium 109
Sorbolene cream 91, 111
soups 30-1
spaghetti bolognaise 132
spicy foods 39, 88, 113
spring 27, 114-16
St John's wort 72
'standardised extract' 154-5
steroid cream 86, 93
stomach-aches and upsets 66, 70, 96-8, 127
stress 67, 74-5, 128
sugar 71, 108, 118
sugar cravings 120, 123
sugar levels 50
summer 109-10
Summer Delight herbal tea 128-9
sunblock 109
sunshine 94
supper ideas 141
supplements
  buying 153-6
sweets 118
swimming 33, 93-4, 149
swollen glands 10
symptoms, as used in this book 6

tannin 104
tea *see* black tea; herbal teas
teeth, cleaning 149-50
television 54, 76, 118
temperatures 17-18
threadworms 150
thrush 147-8
Thuja 23
thumb-sucking 146
toilet hygiene 148
tonics 73, 110 *see also* particular problems
tonsillitis 9, 36, 42-7
toxins 65
treats 62, 74
Triple E herbal tea 129

urinary tract infections 121, 149

vaccination 22-3
vagina, inflamed 147-8
vaporisers 40
vegetables 13, 90, 98
vegetarian diet 29-30
Ventolin 33
vervain 78
Vicks inhaler 40
viral infection 20
viruses 9
vitamin A 11, 23, 94
vitamin Bs 52, 63, 81
vitamin C 12, 19, 39, 51, 111
vitamin D 94

watermelon 17
wax in the ears 36, 37, 42
weight control 117-30
wheat 25, 28, 122
white blood cells 9, 12
white flour 12
winter 112-14
worms 150

zinc 13
zinc cream 109